NUGGETS
FROM THE
GOLDEN AGE OF MEDICINE
NO RELATIONSHIP TO MONEY

KENNETH CHARLES BAGBY, M.D.

outskirts
press

NUGGETS FROM THE GOLDEN AGE OF MEDICINE
No Relationship to Money
All Rights Reserved.
Copyright © 2017 Kenneth Charles Bagby, M.D.
v10.0

The opinions expressed in this manuscript are solely the opinions of the author and do not represent the opinions or thoughts of the publisher. The author has represented and warranted full ownership and/or legal right to publish all the materials in this book.

This book may not be reproduced, transmitted, or stored in whole or in part by any means, including graphic, electronic, or mechanical without the express written consent of the publisher except in the case of brief quotations embodied in critical articles and reviews.

Outskirts Press, Inc.
http://www.outskirtspress.com

ISBN: 978-1-4787-8626-9

Cover Photo © 2017 thinkstockphotos.com. All rights reserved - used with permission.

Outskirts Press and the "OP" logo are trademarks belonging to Outskirts Press, Inc.

PRINTED IN THE UNITED STATES OF AMERICA

PREFACE

NUGGETS FROM THE GOLDEN YEARS OF MEDICAL PRACTICE IN RURAL NEBRASKA
[The word 'golden' has nothing to do with money.]

I GRADUATED FROM medical school in 1960 and retired 45 years later in 2005. I truly believe that I learned more about medicine, especially the art of the practice of medicine, after graduation than I ever learned in medical school. One medical school professor commented in class, "All that we can really hope to teach you here, during these four years, is enough to keep you out of trouble—the rest is up to you." Much was learned in doctor's lounges during internship and residency days listening to other doctors' medical stories of unusual cases and events. That same sort of learning continued via interaction with colleagues throughout my entire career. The most important message in this entire book, I will state now, and I will repeat on the last page. It has truly been an HONOR to have been allowed to be included in some the most joyous—and in some of the most difficult times in the lives of my patients and their families. In my retirement years, especially since the advent of Obamacare, doctors all over the nation are spending more time with their computers and less time actually talking to their patients. I have often been reminded by my younger colleagues who are still in practice that I was lucky to have practiced medicine during "The Golden Years." That term has nothing to do with money, but rather freedom and TIME to practice medicine to the best of our ability. It is my wish that many medical students, as well as their older colleagues, and perhaps those of you who just have an interest in medicine, will find some "nuggets" in these pages. Many of the medical students who heard many of these stories during their junior or senior preceptorship days in our office have encouraged me to put them into print—so here they are, starting with my own family.

I am convinced that there is a special place in heaven for doctors' wives/spouses. The life of a small-town family doctor thrusts a lot of stress upon the family. We were warned in medical school that the practice of medicine is a very demanding mistress. It took me quite a few years before I realized the truth of that statement. The early years presented the challenge of being on call 24/7, until we were able to structure some changes. Our third son, born three years after our arrival in Blair, was three years old before he first called me Daddy; he referred to me as "Car-Car"–associating me with the coming and going of the family automobile. It was then that I began to lobby our group of doctors for an on-call schedule. The senior doctors in the Blair Clinic were all products of the Great Depression of the 1930s. In those days, they had to work hard, putting in long hours just to put food on the table and a roof over their heads. My wife Carole (an RN by training, but by this time a full-time mom) and I shared our passion for the healing profession. I am certain that background as an RN helped to sustain her as the needs of my patients often took precedence over family plans.

We had only one telephone line at home, that is until our daughter became a teenager, when we realized that she had to have her own private line. Sometimes we went out to a restaurant for supper so that we could have some family time together without the interruption of the telephone.

All during my training years, I enjoyed sitting in doctor's lounges and hearing stories about the unusual events that had happened in my mentors' practices. Just as Hippocrates taught, I learned much about the art and practice of medicine at such times. A few years ago, Carole and I had the opportunity to visit the Greek Island of Kos and sit under the plane tree where Hippocrates taught his students. In my library I have a leaf from that plane tree pressed between the pages of Hippocrates' writings.

It is my hope that some future medical practitioners may glean a nugget or two from the stories that are related in this book. Specific names are omitted or changed. There are a few times in which I use real names, with permission—because of the deep respect that I still hold for those individuals. These stories are about the reality of everyday rural medicine, with a focus on the humor and the successes. I've set them in some loose groupings, but have not tried to impose a strict order. My partner, Dr. Leslie Grace, once said to me, "What I like most about being a doctor in a small town is that there is almost never any such thing as a routine day. Anything at all can happen, and it often does." Being able to step up each new day and meet that challenge is gratifying.

I am reminded of a saying: "The older I get, the better I was." That sounds like something Mark Twain would have said, but Google says otherwise. Every once in a while, the Good Lord will throw in a healthy dose of humility, and His forgiveness is always there. These were the "Golden Years of Medicine"—i.e., free from the intrusions of the federal government that have changed the practice of medicine into the more corporate-like structure that exists today. Enjoy the read.

K. Charles Bagby, M.D.

TABLE OF CONTENTS

Preface	i
Biographical Sketch	1
The Internship Years	9
Clinical Obstetrics In Private Practice	13
Penicillin	27
More Penicillin Miracles	29
Memorable House Calls	31
Unusual Emergencies	33
Lightning	37
A Snowmobile Accident	38
Motorcycles	38
An Accident-Prone Family	40
A Very Rare Event	40
Myasthenia Gravis	41
Another Extremely Rare Illness	41
Jury Duty	43
Constipation In The Elderly,	
Caused By A Parathyroid Adenoma	45

The Value Of Surrounding Yourself With Good People	47
Dr. Richard Gentry	48
Dr. Howard Hunt	51
Dr. Hans Rath	53
An Encounter With Jimsonweed Poisoning	57
Courage: "Soldier On"	59
The Evolution Of Rescue Squads	65
Unusual Presentation Of Pernicious Anemia And Tetanus	69
Tetanus	70
The House With A Red Lantern Over The Door	73
Alcohol-Related Stories	75
The Major Stroke That Was Stopped In Its Tracks	79
Oranges And Eggs: Memories Of Dr. Rudolph Schenken	83
Perceptions About The Practice Of Medicine Over The Span Of My Career	85
Final Comments	89

BIOGRAPHICAL SKETCH

My parents were products of the Great Depression of the 1930s. They were married in 1932 and I was born in 1934. Those were tough economic years for a young married couple to start a life together, let alone a family. My mother told me that the reason I was an only child was that she had a difficult home delivery (I was breech), and that July day was 104 degrees in western Nebraska. My mother and father just decided then and there: that was enough. I turned out to be a normal little boy growing up. I had a wonderful companion, my Boston Bull Terrier named Duke. We lived across the street from the Cheyenne County Courthouse in Sidney, Nebraska. The courthouse was set in the middle of a square block of lush green grass. Several neighborhood boys about my age and I had lots of fun playing cowboys and Indians and football on that seemingly vast expanse of lawn.

I probably did not have a serious thought in my head until I was about nine or ten years old. Then one summer day, I decided to ride my bicycle to the high school to play tennis with some of my friends. I never got to the high school. I had carefully ridden my bicycle along the curb of the street in front of our house. Just before I reached the corner, I heard a loud crash to my left. As I looked to the left, I saw a car racing directly for me—BACKWARDS—and only an arm's length away. I have absolutely no memory of what happened next, until after I landed on the front lawn of the house on that corner, about 15 feet from the street. Two cars had collided at that intersection, throwing one of them into reverse gear, and taking direct aim on me. Hearing the crash, my mother came running out of our house just as I was dusting myself off. My bicycle was crushed underneath that car as it came to rest partially over the curbing. I never made it to the tennis courts. I have never understood how I got off that bicycle, and 10 to 15 feet away from that car without any injury whatsoever. It was as if a guardian angel delivered me out of harm's way. The longer I have lived, the more I believe that is exactly what happened.

In retrospect, after that event I began to focus more clearly on the future. By the time I entered high school, I had become convinced that I wanted to become a Methodist minister. I studied very hard to get good grades, but I also wanted to become an athlete—which took a lot of effort. I was more gangly and clumsy than muscular and graceful in those early to mid-teen years. As such, I had to learn to deal with some occasional bullying. I went out for basketball in the eighth grade. I played some, and occasionally made a basket—but mostly I had to learn to get out of the way of my own feet. As a high school freshman I went out for both football and basketball. I made the starting five on the freshman basketball team. I was still clumsy, so I often fouled out. In the process, a lot of those foul calls went my way and I got to shoot a lot of free throws—and I made most of them. I was awarded the free throw medal at the end of my freshman year.

My freshman football coach was a mild-mannered teacher by the name of Ray Maley. He took me aside one day and told me that he thought I could become a pretty good football player if I could just get "mad" once in a while. I had to think about that for a while. I finally decided that he did not mean angry, but rather more focused and intense. Anyway, one day during my freshman year, the slob who had verbally bullied me on and off for the previous couple of years confronted me in the hallway, directly in front of the high school principal's office. Through clenched teeth, and with a clenched fist he said, "I think that you're a sissy." Suddenly, I felt an inner strength as I stared him in the eyes, and casually and calmly said, "You know, I really do not care what YOU think." *I calmly turned and walked away.* I could see that that response so surprised him, that he did not know how to deal with it. He also turned and walked away, never to bother me again, that I know about. There was another incident either later that year or early the next year, in which someone sitting behind me in assembly hall pressed a lighted cigarette onto the back of my neck. It hurt badly, but boy, did I surprise whoever did that! I did not react, I did not flinch, I did not utter a sound, and I did not even turn around—absolutely no response. I just restrained myself because I believed that that was the way that Jesus wanted me to behave. My guiding principle was, "Turn the other cheek."

Vergal Winn, a valued high school math teacher and basketball referee, taught me not to react if a foul was called on me in a basketball game. Mr. Winn told me, "When you throw up your arms and stomp away after the foul call, I know you well enough to realize that you are blaming yourself for the foul. But all of those people out there in the stands do not know that. They just think you are a poor sport." Later in life, I discovered that my adult hero, Tom Osborne, often gave the same message to his football team as a means of avoiding costly and sometimes unwarranted penalties on the football field.

As a senior I was named to the Scottsbluff Star-Herald's All Western Nebraska honor football team. I went out for the track team for four years, but my purpose was to keep in good physical shape for football and basketball. Finally, my senior year I lettered even though I had no talent for track and field. I taught myself to run the high hurdles and finish the race without knocking any of them over. That was good enough to earn me the fourth spot on the 240-yard high hurdles relay team.

Other extra-curricular activities included playing clarinet in the band for 4 years, and serving as our representative to Cornhusker Boys' State during my junior year. In my senior year I was class president and valedictorian. The most important thing was that the Lord helped me to believe that with His help, I could do anything that was set before me.

The next challenge was college. I had received a Regents scholarship from the University of Nebraska and more from other schools, but I wanted to be a Methodist minister, so I got on a Greyhound bus with my two big suitcases and headed for Nebraska Wesleyan University—about 360 miles from my home in Sidney. I arrived in Lincoln in time to report for preseason football practice. Classes started two weeks later, just after the Labor Day holiday. My first two years in college were spent as a theology major studying the social sciences and religion. I also played linebacker and center on the football team. A major ankle injury, and then reconstructive surgery on my nose, which had been broken during my sophomore year in high school, derailed my athletic ambitions.

As I started doing local preaching in small Lincoln area rural churches during my sophomore year, I began to feel less and less comfortable with the thought of doing that for a lifetime. My grade average during those first two college years was a B. I knew that I was a better student than that because in high school I took every math and science course that our school offered, and my grades were straight A's. My college roommate, Bob Jewett, and our theology professor, Ed Mattingly, helped me to understand that my talents perhaps were better suited for the sciences. I learned that Nebraska Wesleyan had an excellent pre-medicine program that was well respected by area medical schools. I also noticed that most of the pre-med students were among the leading students on campus.

After much consideration and a trip home to talk with my folks, I changed majors from theology to pre-medicine. Actually, the philosophies of both endeavors blend quite well.

I needed one summer school session at the University of Nebraska to pick up a required basic college chemistry course. After that summer, the next two years at Wesleyan were crammed with the scientific courses which, in a normal college class load, would require three years. I was able to graduate from Wesleyan in a total of four years (much to my parents' delight) with the Silver Medal—academically second in my class. I also was elected to Phi Kappa Phi, the small college equivalent of Phi Beta Kappa. My studies at Nebraska Wesleyan prepared me to enter the freshman class at the University Of Nebraska Medical Center in Omaha in 1956.

Switching majors not only changed my future career, it changed my life in an even more important way. I started my junior year at Wesleyan taking basic science courses. I found myself surrounded by new freshman students in a basic biology class where I met my future wife, Carole. She was taking pre-nursing classes with the goal of becoming a registered nurse. That meeting is an interesting story. Carole likes to say that we met in biology lab over a dead frog. I remember it a bit differently.

Next to me was seated (thank you to our Chinese lady professor, Dr. Hsu) an attractive freshman coed. I leaned over and whispered to her, "You probably do not remember me, but I certainly remember your mother's cinnamon rolls!" That proved to be a great line. Two years previously, following a Nebraska Wesleyan Concert Band performance in her hometown, her brother John, a college classmate of mine, had invited a number of the band members to come over to his home after the concert for treats. I had seen Carole in the kitchen helping her mother serve homemade cinnamon rolls. I never will forget how delicious those cinnamon rolls were. Both of us still enjoy sharing a good cinnamon roll. We have never found any as good as her mother's.

I gave Carole an engagement ring on Easter Sunday about two months before I graduated from college. Carole still nudges me when I mention that Easter was on April 1st that year.

We planned to be married a year later, after I finished my first year of medical school in Omaha, and after she finished her first year at Nebraska Methodist Hospital School of Nursing, also in Omaha. However, we found that the training for each of those professions was more time consuming than we had anticipated. I truly lost contact with the real world around me during those four years. I have to remind myself that those were the Eisenhower presidential years. All I can recall of the politics of that era was the start of the interstate highway systems. Carole and I found that we had almost no time to see each other. We wanted to at least talk to each other every day. There were no cell phones in 1956, and dorms had only one telephone per floor. Too much time was wasted waiting in line to make a telephone call to a phone line that was almost always busy anyway. So, we decided to move the wedding date up to December 18, the start of our mutual two-week Christmas vacation from classes. We knew that the timing complicated plans for both families. We were very grateful that everyone rallied to help. Everything worked out well, as we got to see each other, and we could both give our medical studies the attention that was needed.

Carole was a freshman in nursing school in 1956, and in that era, she needed special permission from Miss Fagan, the director of her nursing school, to get married. We went together to see Miss Fagan. Since Carole was academically first in her class, and I passed muster, we were given permission with one provision. If she were to become pregnant before the last five months of nursing school, she would have to drop out.

Our first son, David, was born in December 1959, seven months after Carole graduated and received her RN degree, and also her Bachelor of Science degree from Nebraska Wesleyan. I had only a few months left before I received my M.D. degree.

There are a number of memorable moments that occurred during medical school days, and during the internship that followed. Early in my senior year of medical school, on my first night on emergency room call for the pediatric department at the University of Nebraska Medical Center, I was the first one to examine a two-week-old infant, who had a high fever of about 105. He was extremely irritable. Just touching this infant, especially when moving his hips and legs, elicited that remarkable bug-eyed facial expression described in the textbooks, accompanied by screams of pain. I recalled reading in the textbook about the clinical presentation of meningitis in children, and how much this case resembled that. I called the on-call pediatric resident and told him that I thought this child had meningitis. He replied, "Well, I doubt that, but I will come and take a look anyway." After he examined the baby, he said that he still doubted that diagnosis, but since I had mentioned it, we should do the diagnostic spinal tap anyway. When the opalescent (cloudy) spinal fluid appeared from the needle, he exclaimed, "Oh my God, you're right!" Subsequent gram stain and culture proved that it was meningococcal meningitis, a highly contagious and often fatal type of meningitis. Prompt hospitalization and proper treatment with penicillin saved the baby's life. All of the emergency room contacts were required to take prophylactic antibiotics. The chairman of the pediatric department complimented me, and I got an "A" for the course.

My last clinical rotation before graduation was my Senior Preceptorship. I spent a six-week stint in the office of Doctors Bert Pyle and Sam Perry in Gothenburg, Nebraska. Gothenburg was then a town with a population of about 3,000 or so people located in central Nebraska. Conveniently, U.S. Highway 30 passed through the town about one block away from the clinic. One day, into the office walked–rather gingerly–a British Army Sergeant who was in the process of hiking across the United States from the Pacific to the Atlantic Oceans. We had already read about this journey in the Omaha World-Herald. He announced in a very British accent, "I got a painful pile." It was then that I learned how to take care of a painful, thrombosed hemorrhoid. Dr. Pyle examined him as I looked over his shoulder. With the aid of some iodine, local anesthetic, and a scalpel blade the thrombosed hemorrhoid was evacuated of the offending blood clot. After a few instructions to the sergeant and his entourage about how to care for him for a few days, he was sent on his way to New York City. The newspaper later reported that he completed his journey successfully.

THE INTERNSHIP YEARS

AFTER GRADUATION FROM medical school, I elected to remain in Omaha for a one-year rotating internship, which in those days was required of every new graduate. Any specialty training would follow that internship year. I chose Nebraska Methodist Hospital where my wife was already working, having earned her RN degree the previous year. We already lived in an apartment just one block west of the Methodist Hospital on Cuming Street, making an address change unnecessary.

The first day on the Surgery service of my internship at Methodist presented me with a challenge. One of the first patients on early morning intern rounds that day was a young lady who had had abdominal surgery a couple of days before. She was gassy, distended and had generalized abdominal pain. Suspecting a possible small bowel obstruction, I ordered an x-ray of her abdomen. When I went to the radiology department to view the x-ray, there was a surgical sponge that had been inadvertently left behind from her surgery. When I informed her surgeon of the problem, he found a graceful way to take her back to surgery and correct the problem.

The Internal Medicine service: One day I worked up and recorded a history and physical exam for a new patient who had been admitted by one of our local attending physicians. I recorded in my differential diagnosis that I suspected that she was pregnant. When I was making my intern rounds the next morning, I was surprised to find that she was already downstairs in surgery, undergoing a hysterectomy. I rushed downstairs, and as I entered the surgery changing room, I heard Dr. Rudy Schenken, the chief of pathology at Methodist, literally plastering this surgeon to the wall for taking out the uterus—which contained a small fetus inside. All hell broke loose over that episode.

Another patient that I saw on that same internal medicine rotation had been admitted by one of the internal medicine specialists. This patient was having blood pressure and breathing problems. I noticed that his frequent blood pressure recordings indicated a very narrow pulse pressure, i.e., the systolic and the diastolic blood pressure had become so close together that at times they seemed almost the same. I called the internist, and suggested that we should maybe consider that the patient might have a cardiac tamponade. He agreed, and he called our chest/cardiovascular surgeon, Dr. Delbert Neis. With the aid of fluoroscopy, he inserted a long needle into the pericardial sac which surrounds the heart, and removed the bloody fluid that was squeezing the heart muscle and severely limiting his cardiac output. The patient was immediately relieved. The internist commented to me after that episode, "If you should ever want to enter an internal medicine residency, I would be glad to help you." That did a lot to raise my confidence level.

One morning on the obstetrical service I was called to see one of the newborns in the nursery. He was very spitty and could not seem to hold down his formula. I thought that I should try to pass a nasogastric tube to clean out the mucous in his stomach. The tube would not go down, only curling up in his mouth instead. The baby was born with incomplete development of his esophagus—and thus no connection from his throat to his stomach. We called the chest surgeon who repaired this case of esophageal atresia that very afternoon. The baby did well following corrective surgery.

The following is one of my most memorable experiences during my internship. One day while on the obstetrical service, a lady who was pregnant with her sixth child was admitted by her family doctor. This lady was not in labor, but was near her due date. She had delivered all of her previous five babies at home. Her labors were so short, fast and easy that she could never make it to the hospital in time. This time she was determined to have the sixth baby in a hospital. I also surmised that with five kids at home she needed the rest. So, here she was, waiting. I made sure that the OB nurse would call me the very minute anything started to happen.

After a couple of days of just resting, I was called to her side and she said, "I feel like I am beginning to open up." I could detect no regular contractions. However, we moved her rapidly to the delivery table, got her draped and ready. Then with the aid of retractors (with the mother's permission) to hold the vaginal walls apart, we watched the cervix slowly dilate from about two cm to a full ten cm dilation. We witnessed the slow descent and rotation of the head as it descended past the spines (the narrowest part of the pelvis), then baby's head and neck extend as the baby moved out of the vaginal outlet. Just like time-lapse photography, but all in the course of less than five or so minutes of real time. It was amazing to actually see the process happen like that right in front of our eyes. The mother was totally comfortable throughout the entire event. The birth of a baby is truly a miracle. To this day, I still feel fortunate to have had some small part in this miracle of birth so many times during my career.

One day, during my surgery rotation at Methodist Hospital, there came to the emergency room a gentleman who had an unusual injury. He was using a power drill for a carpentry project and he dropped it. It had only an on/off rocker type power switch, so when he dropped it the motor continued to run. He was seated at the time, so the drill fell into his lap, got tangled up in his light-weight summer clothing, and—you probably have guessed—proceeded to rip open his scrotum, leaving both testicles hanging out in the breeze. I spent the next hour or so helping a plastic surgeon repair the damage in surgery under general anesthesia. The testicles lived on for another day.

    I completed my internship in June of 1961. Two months later, East Germany began building the Berlin Wall, with approval of the Soviet Union. A huge U.S. military buildup followed, and at the age of twenty-seven I was drafted as a doctor into the U.S. Army, with the rank of captain.

CLINICAL OBSTETRICS IN PRIVATE PRACTICE

DURING MY ALMOST 2 years in the military, I had no involvement in taking care of anyone who was sick. All of those patients went to the hospitals where other doctors provided their care. I also had no involvement in surgery or obstetrics during that period of time. I felt like I needed a refresher course in those areas. In those days, there was no such thing as today's three-year family practice residencies. Those didn't evolve in Nebraska until about 1968.

When I left the service in September 1963, Dr. Rudy Schenken arranged for me to return to Methodist Hospital for a year, where he promised to provide for me the refresher experience that I needed, concentrating on surgery and obstetrics. That experience proved to be exactly what I needed for the next 41 years of practice in Blair.

The extra year at Methodist Hospital was a family practice residency, of sorts. A great opportunity presented when I became aware that Drs. Howard, Sievers, and Grace in Blair desperately needed help.

1964 was the year that Dr. Rudy Sievers was president of the Nebraska Medical Association (NMA). He was frequently away from home base attending to NMA responsibilities. Since Dr. Clifford

Howard was semi-retired, that left Dr. Leslie Grace to carry the heaviest load of the practice. He had to work long, hard hours just to handle the increase in the patient load in addition to caring for his own patients and his usual duties to oversee the business functions of the office. At that time there was no office manager, except for Pat Nelson, who managed the front desk and receptionists.

Dr. Sievers and Dr. Howard both entered medical school at Nebraska in 1932. Rudy Sievers' father sold a farm and put the money in the bank to help pay for Rudy's medical education. The Great Depression hit and the banks went broke, leaving Rudy with no money. It took him eight years to finish medical school. He raised money by waiting tables and doing research for drug companies. He graduated with two degrees, his M.D. and a Ph.D. in Pharmacology. Dr. Sievers then spent the WWII years in Washington, D.C., working at the National Institutes of Health.

Clifford Howard did some barbering on the side to pay for his medical education. He opened his private practice in Blair in the late 1930s. He rented space on the second story of a downtown business building, as did many doctors in that era of the '30s and '40s. He and another physician were the only M.D.s in Blair during WWII. Each one maintained separate offices.

After the war, Rudy returned to Blair and joined with his former classmate Cliff Howard to form the Blair Clinic. In conjunction with a dentist, Dr. Ehlers, they built the first ground-level Blair Clinic near 16th and Lincoln St. in downtown Blair. After Leslie Grace, M.D. joined them in the mid-1950s, they found the existing building too cramped, and began discussing building a new Blair Clinic on land next door to the new Blair hospital, which had opened its doors to patients in 1956. Dr. Howard was semi-retired and did not want to participate financially in the new building, but agreed to rent space there until he fully retired. Dr. Sievers and Dr. Grace and their wives formed the Blair Clinic Building Corporation, with the legal assistance of attorney Roy I. Anderson.

They then proceeded to take out a mortgage and buy the land and build the new Blair Clinic. That new building was built in 1963 with room for four doctors. In 1964, that fourth doctor proved to be me. Three empty rooms were available, for which I had to purchase the furnishings. I remembered that in medical school we were advised to buy the largest desk that we could fit into our office. I did that, plus chairs, and a big bookcase. At first I only purchased enough furniture for one exam room. However, after two months, I was busy enough that I had to furnish the second exam room. All of the doctors paid the same rent, including the original two investors.

The finances of the Blair Clinic were somewhat unusual. Each doctor maintained his own practice, but we shared expenses such as salaries for our employees, utilities, lawn care, etc. The finances were kept separate, and the money was allocated separately. It was a complicated system. In other words, the harder you worked, the higher was your net income. If you did not want to work hard, your net income reflected that. We were all happy with that arrangement.

Rent at the Blair Clinic was paid monthly by each individual doctor. It was a bit of a shock to me when I discovered that the first month's rent was due in ADVANCE. I managed somehow. After several years I was invited to become a full partner by purchasing an equal share of the new Blair Clinic at a price equal to what Dr. Sievers and Dr. Grace had already invested. It took me a number of years to pay back that debt, but it was well worth it.

Dr. Grace delivered a lot of babies in those days. For the first couple of decades after I joined the Blair Clinic, our local hospital handled about 200-plus obstetrical cases per year. Those numbers were split almost 50/50 between Dr. Grace and myself. As the next two decades went by, those obstetrical numbers dwindled for both of us. Dr. Grace also was quite good with orthopedics. He was very helpful to me, a young Doc just learning to run my own practice when I first came to Blair.

From the mid-1960s until the early 1990s, I delivered about 90 to 110 babies every year. That actually is more than some OB specialists delivered in the big city. On two separate occasions I delivered four babies for four different mothers in the same 24-hour period, and on one of those occasions none of those mothers were in labor at the same time. I also had two occasions where two deliveries happened simultaneously. Obviously I could not be in two places at once, so this was a time when your partners stepped in to help.

One February I was the attending physician for 28 deliveries. I felt like a walking zombie at the end of that month due to lack of sleep. In my career, I delivered 13 sets of twins, all of them full term and healthy. None of the twins weighed less than six pounds. I never delivered triplets.

Most deliveries are normal and everyone is overjoyed. However, obstetrics is one area of the practice of medicine where what seems normal can evolve into a horrendous emergency in the blink of an eye. Whether it is a prolapsed umbilical cord, or massive bleeding from a placenta previa (an edge of the placenta presenting first at the opening of the cervix), or an abruption (early separation of the placenta, which causes bleeding inside of the uterus while the baby is still in there), immediate action is required, often a cesarean section delivery.

One such case I shall never forget. This young mother was in labor with her first baby. Contractions were vigorous but progress was very slow. I spent the night at the hospital watching her progress and talking with her husband. Slowly she became fully dilated, and it became apparent that her vigorous pushing was not bringing the baby's head down well, so she needed some assistance with forceps. I had worked at Methodist with Dr. Jim Kovarik, who was a magician with forceps. What I learned from him proved to be invaluable in the years to come.

At any rate, we went into the delivery room where I administered a saddle block anesthetic, a common procedure in the 1970s. A saddle block involves injection of an anesthetic low in the spinal canal where it is intended to block the pain nerves to the pelvic muscles that are being stretched in the birthing process. Within a minute or two, the patient suddenly exclaimed, "I cannot breathe." A simultaneous uterine contraction had forced the anesthetic upward in the spinal canal, instead of letting it settle to the bottom as it was supposed to do.

Instead it paralyzed the muscles that she used to breathe. Fortunately, it was 9 a.m. on a Saturday morning, and every single doctor on the medical staff was making rounds at the moment that I called a code blue for the delivery room, as the patient and baby crashed. Their lives were in immediate danger. Everyone leaped into action. One doctor started chest compressions; another took an anesthesia mask and pumped oxygen into her lungs. Within minutes we had completed a cesarean section. As soon as the baby was out of the uterus, the mother began responding like any other post-op cesarean section patient. Unfortunately, the baby sustained neurologic damage and died at the university hospital a few days later. The sequel to this story: almost exactly one year later I delivered, by scheduled cesarean section, a healthy girl for this couple. For many years later, although they did not live in Blair any more, I would see the husband periodically. He would proudly show me the pictures of his beautiful daughter, and later on, her younger siblings in their growing family.

I subsequently found an article in the New England Journal of Medicine, reporting on two cases at Massachusetts General Hospital (Harvard Medical School's major teaching hospital), which were absolutely identical to this case. Unfortunately, they lost both the mother and the baby in each case. It was the immediate availability of the entire medical staff and their immediate actions that allowed us to have at least saved the mother in this case.

In recent years the evolution of the epidural technique has replaced the saddle block—a much safer procedure for delivery when that type of pain relief is needed.

I remember another obstetrical case in which I have always felt that the Lord was watching over us. I had just completed a routine cesarean section. I forget now the details of the case, except for this: as I was helping to move the mother off the operating room table, she mentioned that she felt some itching, but it passed in a few seconds. At the time I thought little of it. About 15 minutes later however, the itching returned and she broke out in a severe case of hives, became short of breath and started to wheeze. Bingo! – The light bulb in my brain lit up – amniotic fluid pulmonary embolism. This is a very rare complication of cesarean section. Amniotic fluid contains, among other things, "baby poop." If amniotic fluid finds its way into the mother's circulatory system before the muscles of the now empty uterus can clamp down, she can die. I picked up the telephone and talked with my internal medicine colleague. We immediately started this patient on massive doses of IV steroids which saved her life. This is the one and only case of amniotic fluid pulmonary embolism that I encountered in my medical career. I felt the presence of the Lord with that one. How else would the correct diagnosis come to mind instantly, for such a rare problem?

Another memorable cesarean section was to help one of my colleagues. He called me at 6:00 a.m. one morning and told me that he was delivering twins. The first twin had actually precipitated in bed without his help. However, the placenta had only partially separated, and had trapped the second baby in the fundus (body) of the uterus. Meanwhile, bleeding from the uterus was profuse. We had to get that second baby out of there as fast as we could, and cesarean section was the only way. I received the call at home at 6 a.m.–the healthy baby was born by cesarean section at 6:30 a.m. We had to brag a bit about that one.

In the very early years of my practice in Blair, in the late 1960s, a rare complication occurred. Remember, this was quite a few years before the era of fetal ultrasound. During a routine prenatal exam at about seven months gestation, I began to notice a hard lump in the fundus of the uterus. This lump grew rapidly, until it became quite large. Suspicious, I ordered an X-ray. What we found was a baby with a huge hydrocephalus–and it was lying in the breech presentation. I consulted with an obstetrician, and we were convinced that cesarean section was the only possible means of delivery, as the head was already much too big to pass through the birth canal. After discussion with mother, father and all concerned, we performed the cesarean section. The baby was born alive, with a greatly enlarged head, confirming what we had seen on the x-ray, but died after just a few minutes. Now, in more modern times, early intervention with intrauterine surgical techniques hopefully could result in a better outcome.

Sometimes, obstetrical cases expose the deficiencies of our society, and present what at times seems to be an unsolvable dilemma. As this next story unfolds, you may realize that this poor family needed all of the sympathy and help that we could muster. At first this unfortunate, uneducated lady was irritating to me because she always presented in the late evening or the middle of the night with a problem that needed prompt attention. But as her many problems continued to unfold, I came to realize that even though her husband worked at a low-skilled job, they were as poor as church mice. They had no automobile so she had to depend upon other people for transportation, as they lived about 20+ miles away from Blair.

One evening after a hard day in the office, I received a telephone call from the emergency room nurse at the hospital. It seems that they had this lady who was experiencing severe pain in her rectum. She felt she had to have a bowel movement, but just could not. On examination, she was pregnant and ready to deliver. She also had an umbilical hernia that enlarged to the size of a volleyball with each contraction. She delivered a healthy, normal baby, and the hernia was greatly reduced. She said, yes, she noticed that she had not had a period for a few months, but she did not know why. After about three or four days in the hospital, and with all of the education that we could give her, she and the baby went home. She was given instructions to return for follow-up care for the both of them.

She never returned until late one night, about a year later, I got a call at home from the emergency room nurse about a lady who had a lot of rectal pain. You guessed it, here she was again about ready to have another baby. Only this time she was hypertensive, toxemic, and sadly, delivered a dead baby. All she could think about was, "I got to have another one"—she said, over and over.

Toxemia of pregnancy is a complication in which the normal mechanisms that control blood pressure go haywire, and can even result in death of the mother and/or the baby. This is a primary reason why good, regular prenatal care is so important.

I finally got her blood pressure under control. She actually returned to the office several times, until a few months later, she showed up in our emergency room about midnight with an acute bowel obstruction. Dr. Rath arrived promptly and we operated in the middle of the night. The entire right colon had become strangulated in that huge umbilical hernia. We removed her right colon, repaired the umbilical hernia, and—guess what?—her uterus was enlarged. She was about four months pregnant with her third baby.

From this point on, the previous umbilical hernia repair broke down before the next delivery, then another pregnancy, etc., etc. After several babies, including the one stillbirth, and three related bowel obstructions–all with large sections of strangulated (dead) bowel that had to be removed, as well as re-repairs of the recurrent umbilical hernia–she was running out of bowel. We feared another pregnancy could bring fatal complications. After some discussion, she chose to have her fallopian tubes tied.

As the kids were getting older, the school nurse sent one of them home. The Burt–Washington County Home Health Association was becoming organized and funded in the area in that time. I sent the home health nurses out to follow up. The nurse reported sadly that they did not have mattresses on which to sleep. The association was able to help this family a lot. They needed all the help that we could muster.

During the late 1960s, I was approached by an Omaha area mother whose teenage daughter had become pregnant. The mother did not want to send her daughter away to another part of the country for six months or more, as some families did in those days. For privacy reasons, the girl's mother asked if I could deliver the baby in the Blair hospital, and see her at our clinic for the necessary prenatal visits, after dark when the only ones around were the mother, daughter and myself. I agreed—only if they would visit first with a good adoption agency, which I arranged. The pregnancy and delivery were uneventful. At the postpartum exam, both mother and the baby were doing well. Then the adoption agency took over from there.

Most of the babies that I delivered were in the hospital.

One was at home—the baby came very fast, fortunately, I was able to get to the home before the rescue squad arrived. I also delivered one baby in the front seat of an automobile—in the parking lot of our hospital. Prior to the 1950s, many deliveries occurred at home. One of the best stories about home deliveries that I ever heard was told by one of my senior partners, Dr. Clifford Howard. He was attending a patient at home here in Blair. The mother was a large woman, and when he entered the bedroom she was sitting on the chamber pot. She promptly dropped a baby into the pot. Dr. Howard helped get her off of the pot and back into bed. After he retrieved the infant and was wiping the baby clean, the mother got back on the pot and dropped in another baby. Dr. Howard proudly walked into the hospital carrying two babies (pretty well cleaned up) in his arms. Both babies did well.

The smallest baby that I delivered weighed one pound and twelve ounces. He fit nicely in the palm of my hand. For some unknown reason, the mother went into labor two and one-half months early. The year was about 1970, a few years before the first neonatal intensive care unit was established in this part of the country at the University of Nebraska Medical Center in Omaha. Thanks to the almost constant care of our experienced nurses, including Kittie Stricklett and Margaret Laughlin, this baby not only survived, but thrived in our nursery in Blair. We had a nice (for those days) isolette. The baby was tube fed a few cc's of special preemie formula every hour, but it was mostly the tender, loving care of Kittie and Margaret, and of our staff of devoted nurses, that brought that baby through with flying colors. We were indeed fortunate that the baby did not have any lung problems. The baby weighed right at five pounds when he was dismissed from our hospital at age four months. He is now a career staff sergeant in the U.S. Army. His mother keeps us updated.

The largest baby that I delivered weighed 11 pounds, 10½ ounces. Both mother and father were plus-sized persons. No problems occurred with the delivery.

Not every story has a happy ending. One such episode happened one evening when I had to step in to deliver a baby for another doctor who happened to be unavailable. Having never seen the patient before, I introduced myself before examining her to determine just where we were in the course of her active labor. What I felt was disturbing, because the presenting part was irregular and lumpy—unlike anything I had ever felt before. This was in the days before ultrasound had been invented. I told the parents that I thought a flat film x-ray of the abdomen would be helpful to guide the course of delivery.

What I saw was shocking—the baby was anencephalic. This means that although the facial bones and eyes were present, there was no skull, and therefore no brain above the level of the eyes. I showed this x-ray to the father, and then we both had to prepare to tell the mother about the problem. Of course the baby did not live. For some reason this had not been detected in her prenatal visits with her physician. The delivery room was very quiet and weepy during that delivery. My heart went out to this couple who had to bear such a terrible burden of such an extremely rare anomaly. The real miracle of birth is that everything goes right most of the time.

It was such a special privilege to supervise the birth of so many healthy babies. One of my greatest pleasures was to observe these same children as they grew up. I enjoyed going to school plays, concerts, and athletic events and watching the kids whom I had delivered perform. Even now in retirement, I frequently have a grown, middle-aged man or woman come up to me and say, "Do you remember me? You delivered me." One day, at a Nebraska State Medical Association meeting, I had the occasion to sit down for lunch with Dr. McGoogan. Dr. Mac was my OB professor in Medical School. He was perhaps the most respected of all Omaha obstetricians, actively delivering babies at age 80. He delivered babies for the spouses of many of the medical students. He said that he had the same experiences with obstetrics that I did. He liked to go to the medical school graduations and count the number of graduates for whom he personally presided at their birth.

During my last 10 years in practice I was happy to see the younger doctors in our practice take over the bulk of the obstetrical work. My aging body just could not endure the night time hours that are so often required. The last baby that I delivered was by special request. As it turned out, we had enough warning with false labor contractions that the father, who was out of the country on business, was able to board an airplane and arrive back in Blair in time for the birth. After he arrived, I started a Pitocin IV drip. The delivery and birth were entirely normal.

Another story comes to mind. This is one of the complications with which one must deal when you practice obstetrics. Late one evening near midnight, I was at the hospital, having just finished a delivery. I received a telephone call from one the obstetrical specialists who

I knew in the general Omaha area. The specialist had a patient who was having symptoms of a miscarriage. The patient had asked her obstetrician to transfer her to my care in Blair, as I was well known to her family. So—the obstetrician called me to explain the case and asked if I would accept the transfer. I agreed. As I was already on my way home, I left orders with the nurse to call me at home when the patient arrived, which turned out to be somewhere between 2 and 3 a.m. At that time she was stable, had minimal cramping and almost no bleeding, and was comfortable. I instructed the nurse to keep a close watch and to call if there were any change, and I went back to sleep.

The next morning when I arrived at the hospital, I took this patient to our emergency room where I could do an adequate examination. While I was doing the pelvic examination, she suddenly went into shock. Obviously, a tubal pregnancy had just ruptured. Our general surgeon, Dr. Rath, was just finishing a short, early case in the operating room down the hall. I started IVs in both arms and as the lab was preparing blood for transfusion, we got her into the operating room where we were able to save her life. A pumping artery from the ruptured tubal pregnancy had already filled her abdomen with blood.

I did not learn until later the actual reason why this transfer had occurred. It seems that this obstetrician had delivered this patient's first baby for her several years previously. However, that obstetrical bill had never been paid. So, when this patient called this obstetrician's office about these symptoms, she was told that she could not be seen because of her previous unpaid bills. What did I learn from this case? When a specialist refers a patient to the Family Practice doctor, be a bit leery. There may be more to it than you think.

Thank goodness my surgical colleague, Dr. Rath, was in the hospital when this happened. He told me later that if this ever happened again and he was not on site, just go ahead and open her up and stop the bleeding, and he would get here as fast as he could. I was pleased to have him express that kind of confidence in me. One other time, after I had finished a cesarean section with a substitute anesthetist whose home base was elsewhere, he told me that I did a better cesarean section than the OB specialists with which he usually worked. That helped bolster my confidence.

I kept a little black appointment book in my coat pocket that contained the names of my OB patients, their due dates and their blood type. These were the days before pagers and cell phones, and since I was delivering up to 100 babies a year in those years, I usually had eight or more due every month. I consulted that book before I went anywhere other than home or the hospital, so that the OB nurse knew where to find me. A trip to Omaha would require me to call back a couple of times from a pay phone from somewhere.

One Saturday noon in the 1970s, I was attending a Burt/Washington County Medical Society luncheon at a small roadside restaurant located about halfway between Oakland and Tekamah, Nebraska, normally about an hour's drive from Blair. I received a call at the restaurant from our hospital's OB nurse. I had a mother arrive in early labor. I remembered that her first labor had been easy and fast, and since this second labor probably would be even faster, I jumped in my car and headed for Blair. It is a wide-open stretch of road between Oakland and Tekamah, but I was stopped by a highway patrolman along that stretch. He said that I was doing 80 miles an hour. I did not tell him that a few miles before that I had slowed down considerably *to* the 80-mph mark. Anyway, when I explained my mission, he kindly gave me a speedy escort directly to the Blair hospital, where I arrived just in the nick of time.

PENICILLIN

The miracle of penicillin

―――∽∽―――

One day in my early years of practice a middle-aged lady came to my office. We will call her Grace. Her appearance was rather plain, and she was slender—actually a bit malnourished, it seemed. Her clothing was clean but worn and a bit frayed. She had come to see me about her swollen hemorrhoids. She obviously had considerable pain, but her affect was strange with an almost giddy type of giggle when she answered questions, somewhat inappropriately it seemed. The mainstay of treatment of painful, prolapsed hemorrhoids is the generous use of Sitz baths (one spends as much time as possible sitting in a tub of warm water which feels Oh So Good). This presented a major obstacle in the treatment of Grace's hemorrhoids, since she lived in a home in Blair with no indoor plumbing. This was in the late 1960s, and her home was perhaps the only remaining home within the Blair city limits that still had no indoor plumbing. A lack of funds or insurance led her to refuse hospitalization. She and I managed to find some way to treat and resolve her hemorrhoid problem, although it did require several visits to the office. Each time she left the office I also noticed that as she left the exam room and walked down the rather narrow hallway, she seemed to bounce off both walls with a slightly wide-based gait.

Within a few months of the resolution of her hemorrhoid problem, Grace presented to the emergency room of our hospital with a rather nasty displaced ankle fracture. I referred her to an orthopedic specialist friend of mine in Omaha. Grace had to have surgical fixation of the fracture with pins and plates. With a long leg cast and very limited mobility she required some time in the hospital, so several days after her surgery, she was returned to our hospital for that care. The orthopedic specialist mentioned to me on the telephone, "By the way, this lady has a positive serology." Back in those days, some hospitals had medical staff requirements that *every* patient admitted had a few required laboratory tests done on admission. This hospital was one of the last hospitals in Omaha that required a serology blood test for syphilis on every patient. It did not take Medicare and the insurance companies very long put a stop to that practice—no more "routine" tests. However, in Grace's case it was a key. That information prompted me to perform a lumbar puncture. In the few days that it took to get the test results, she rapidly deteriorated mentally and physically. Her speech became very slurred and incoherent, and she became unable to sit upright in bed or wheelchair. She could not feed herself. A positive colloidal gold curve test on her spinal fluid confirmed the diagnosis of neurosyphilis. I proceeded to give her very large doses of penicillin on a daily basis. She progressively improved, regaining slowly her muscle strength and her speech improved enough so that she could converse, feed herself, and she could handle herself well enough after two or three weeks that she could go to a care home.

In those days, nursing homes were not of the quality that they are today. Where Grace went really was a boarding house that offered food, a clean bed and personal care. I continued to see her on a daily basis, and gave her a daily shot of penicillin. By the time her fracture healed, and her cast was removed, she was able to ambulate and go home.

Of course, she still had the Tabes (neurologic damage due to syphilis), and one day a couple of years later she fell, and presented to our hospital with a fracture of her hip. I assisted a different orthopedic surgeon with her hip pinning. Before the surgery, I alerted the surgeon and the entire operative crew that this patient had a diagnosis of neurosyphilis. After the open reduction was accomplished, the next step in the operation is to insert the guide wire through the trochanter, along the neck of the femur and into the femoral head. The fixation pin then slides easily into place over the guide wire. This particular surgical tray mistakenly had on it a Steinman pin, which looks much like the guide wire except that it had a very sharp, spear-like point—unlike the much blunter guide wire. The surgical nurse inadvertently handed the surgeon the Steinman pin. The surgeon, with his left index finger on the femoral neck of the hip bone, as a guide, then inserted the pin, which plunged in too fast and too deep—right though the femoral neck (of the hip bone) and right through the tip of the surgeon's index finger. The surgeon started his own personal course of penicillin therapy within five minutes of the conclusion of that operation. The patient recovered, and lived a few more years before dying of other causes. After some 30 years, the surgeon is now retired—and he walks with a normal gait.

MORE PENICILLIN MIRACLES

One day, in about the 1980s era, there was a young freshman girl from Dana College in Blair who had become ill while in Lincoln attending the state basketball tournament. She had gone to see her high school alma mater play. Because she did not feel well, the group returned directly to Blair. Her condition deteriorated on the way home. Her friends brought her directly to the Blair Clinic. My nurse helped her down the hall, and told me that I needed to see this patient right away. She had a fever of over 104. She hurt all over and was very irritable. We transferred her to the hospital emergency room, just across the parking lot from our clinic. I ordered a stat blood count. A few minutes later the lab called me with the report: her white blood cell count was just short of 30,000, with a 'left shift,' showing a high number of young, immature white blood cells—indicating the bone marrow's response to a severe infection.

I literally ran to the emergency room, where she was lying on a gurney, comatose by now. I performed a spinal tap that revealed the suspected meningococcal meningitis. Then I called my internal medicine friend, Dr. Ron Anderson, who immediately started her on large doses of IV penicillin. She was over the hump and doing well in two or three days.

This type of meningitis is highly contagious, and often it is fatal. All of us who were exposed, including those who rode in the car with her, had to take a course of medicine to prevent us from contracting it also.

MEMORABLE HOUSE CALLS

MY MOST UNUSUAL house call was not to a house, but to a train. My telephone rang late one evening in the mid-1970s or so. I was called to see a gentleman with a bad sore throat. This gentleman was in the caboose of a train which had stopped just across a RR crossing about 1/2 block north of the local Dairy Queen. After I arrived at the Dairy Queen, I walked to the caboose on the track, and some of the train crew helped me aboard. The crewman who was sick had a case of pustular tonsillitis. After checking the usual vital signs, I gave him a shot of penicillin and a prescription to fill after they arrived at the train's destination. After we got him tucked in, I got off of the caboose and the train continued on its way west. He was instructed to check in with his doctor as soon as he arrived home.

Another unusual early-years house call came before the advent of the Blair Rescue Squad. A family who lived about 5 miles west of Blair, near a country crossroads called Orum, called one cold wintery night. They asked if I could make a house call to try to stop their mother's very bad nose bleed. Often times that is a difficult task even in the hospital emergency room. I suggested that they bring her to the hospital. They replied that since she weighed over 350 lbs., the only way they could get her to the hospital was to put her wheelchair in the back of their pickup. Since it was below zero outside that wintery night, I went over to the hospital and borrowed everything that I thought that I might need, including nasal packing, a goose neck lamp and my head mirror, etc. and headed to Orum. I was fortunate that I was able to get the nose packed and stopped the nosebleed, in the home setting. All worked out well.

Another memorable house call was to that same rural crossroads area, on a very cold Sunday afternoon in December. I was headed to a farm home a few miles beyond Orum. Just as I was rounding the corner by the Orum General Store, steam suddenly came out from under the hood of my car. A radiator hose had come off. A family that lived in a nearby home saw what had happened and immediately came to my rescue. The father of the family lifted the hood and said, "I have a radiator hose clamp in my garage—I will be right back." He also had a key to the Orum general store that stood on the other corner of this rural intersection. He returned with a gallon of antifreeze. In less than 15 minutes I was on my way. Now, if I had been in town when this happened on that cold, Sunday afternoon, I would have been in trouble.

UNUSUAL EMERGENCIES

EVERY SMALL-TOWN DOCTOR has stories to tell about the emergencies that arrive on your doorstep requiring immediate decisions and lifesaving action. I can remember several such events. One day our hospital received a call from the Bennington Rescue Squad. Bennington is a community about 15 miles south of Blair. In those days it was rural, but now it is suburban Omaha. They were en route with the nine-year-old daughter of one of my patients. She was reported to be having difficulty breathing.

I met her as she arrived in the emergency room. She was an ashen grey color, clammy, and there was an obvious crowing sound as she struggled to get any air into her lungs. She was in extremis (about ready to die). The diagnosis of acute epiglottis was apparent, and it was obvious to me I had to do something RIGHT NOW to save her life. Within five minutes of the instant that she came through our emergency room door, I had completed a tracheotomy.

I shall never forget the sound of the swish of air that entered her lungs as I made the incision into the trachea. Her skin color immediately changed from the death-like ashen grey to a beautiful rosy pink.

Acute epiglottis is akin to tonsillitis. The function of the flap that we call the epiglottis is to close off the windpipe (trachea) so that food and water go to the stomach and not into the lungs. The tonsil-like tissue near the epiglottis gets infected and swells enough to close off the windpipe. Thus little or no air can get through to the lungs.

A true emergency indeed! That was the one and only tracheotomy that I performed in my entire career. The emergency room crew worked like they had done that same thing every day. Everything went exactly as it had been described to me during my training years. I remember calling a head and neck surgeon friend of mine, later that day, to ask for his guidance about what to do next. I also remember how gratifying it was to see her beautiful wedding photograph in the newspaper some fifteen years later.

A few years later the thought of another emergency tracheotomy crossed my mind briefly. Fortunately it was not needed because the Heimlich maneuver was successful. Carole and I were visiting a rancher cousin who lives deep in the Nebraska Sandhills. My cousin's husband is a cattle rancher who also raised buffalo. We sat down in their kitchen to a wonderful buffalo burger lunch. Suddenly, Marvin started choking and he went to the kitchen sink gagging. As soon as I saw his ears start to turn blue, I rushed over and gave him about three big thrusts of the Heimlich maneuver, before that chunk of meat finally came up. Whew. We all gave a prayer of thanks after we caught our breath.

Another emergency involved a young girl who was about seven or eight years old. The family lived in Fort Calhoun, a small town nine miles south of Blair. The little girl was following behind her father through a doorway. Unaware that his daughter was close behind, he let the glass storm door swing after he passed through. The swinging door caught the child head on and a sharp piece of the shattering glass pierced her armpit. Obviously an artery had been cut, because immediately blood was everywhere. Her father shoved a towel into her armpit to control the bleeding until the rescue squad arrived and took over the armpit pressure. In our emergency room, I asked the squad member to release the pressure just long enough so that I could see what was going on. I had to jump out of the way as a stream of blood shot by my face and hit the wall across the room. Arm pit pressure was resumed immediately and straight to surgery we went, putting surgical garb on the squad member while he continued to apply pressure to the armpit. By the time Dr. Rath arrived we were ready to operate.

He found that the brachial artery, the main artery from the aorta to the right arm, had been completely severed. At that exact spot are also two major branches of the brachial plexus of nerves to the arm, one branch on each side of the severed artery. The nerves were so close to the injury that they were almost adherent to it. Yet, blessedly, there was absolutely no injury to the nerves. Dr. Rath was able to locate both ends of the severed artery, sew them back together, and establish a renewed normal blood flow to the arm. At the end of the procedure the girl had normal pulses in the arm. There was no injury to the brachial plexus of nerves. This was truly one of God's miracles. She made an uneventful recovery with no loss of function. Quick teamwork saved her life and her arm, with the guidance of the Lord.

Dr. Rath was an extremely gifted surgeon. Many times in the old days, instead of dictating an operative report, he would draw an extremely detailed anatomic drawing of what he had just done on the progress note sheet of the patient's chart. A picture is worth a thousand words. He would not be allowed to do that in today's electronic medical record environment. The walls of his home are still covered with oil paint copies of many world class art treasures. He likes to tell the story about his early days in practice, when much of his household furniture consisted of packing crates with a bed sheet or blanket covering them. A visitor commented, "How can you afford all of the Monet paintings on your walls?" They were copies that he had painted.

One day I received a phone call from a local young boy whom I knew well. He had recently been awarded his Eagle Scout badge. He said that he had just been bitten by a black widow spider. I said, "Are you sure?" He replied, "Yes, I have it right here in a glass jar. Do you want to see it?" "You bet," was the answer, "get right over here with it." He had been unpacking a box of bananas at the local grocery store when he was bitten. I immediately put him in the hospital and called our local poison control center in Omaha. They obtained the proper antivenom and a Nebraska State Patrol car was dispatched to bring it to Blair. The antivenom arrived about the time that he was beginning to have systemic symptoms from the bite. He fully recovered, mainly due to the rapid response of our poison control center.

Here is another story about an accident that does not happen every day. This was a gentleman who would often show up in my office, for this and that. This particular time was because he had just shot himself in the shoulder with a bow and arrow. Removal of the arrow was no problem, but my first question was, "How in the world did you manage to do that?" He was attempting to hang a swing from a tree in his yard. Unable to throw a coiled rope over the limb, he resorted to a bow and arrow, with a string tied to the arrow. He intended to tie the rope to the string after he got the arrow over the tree limb. However, on the first try the arrow got entangled in some smaller tree branches. He attempted to retrieve it by tugging on the string. The arrow came right back to him, the point burying itself in his shoulder. He learned not to try that again.

This next story involves a boating accident. Blair is located on the western bank of the Missouri river. One beautiful moonlit summer night, as the hour was approaching midnight, our local rescue squad whistle blew. I was on call for our emergency room. The word was that the rescue squad was bringing in about a dozen people from a boating accident on the river. I called one of my partners for help. While we were awaiting the arrival of the injured, we were informed by the police about what had happened.

A rather large boat had run aground. Unfortunately, when the river channel changed directions, the boat did not. It had slammed into a rock-lined river bank. Smaller boats had to be utilized to remove the injured from the grounded boat, two or three a time, and finally into ambulances. It took several trips by our rescue squad to get all of them off the boat and to our hospital. Meanwhile the triage began and the sun had risen before we got everyone either taken care of here, or transferred to the appropriate hospitals in Omaha. One boater had a head injury that took priority. Other injuries included lacerations and some broken bones. Fortunately, there were no fatalities.

LIGHTNING

One spring evening a young man and his companion decided that it was a nice cool evening to go jogging along a stretch of highway on the north edge of Blair. Our local hospital borders that same stretch of highway. Suddenly a fast-moving rainstorm rolled in, a real gully-washer, with lots of thunder and lightning. After a few minutes it disappeared almost as fast as it came. The rescue squad siren sounded, and my telephone rang—the hospital emergency room nurse said, "Hurry." At an intersection two blocks from the hospital, the storm sewer was overwhelmed and there was a small lake in the street. I tried to plow through but my car stalled. Fortunately there was a local police car on the other side of that lake. The policeman waded out and helped me to his car. As he was taking me to the hospital, I gave him my car keys, and he said, "Don't worry, I will take care of your car." At the emergency room, I encountered a young man who, unfortunately, was dead on arrival. Every hair on his head and chest was singed. After the autopsy, the coroner told me that he could find neither an entry nor an exit wound. That ruled out a direct lightning strike. All that he could say was that there must have been a proximity lightning strike that had caused some sort of cardiac event. The companion, with whom he had been jogging in the rain, was knocked to the ground by the force of that lightning strike. Her jaw was broken as she landed on the pavement, but she had no other injury. This story demonstrates the danger of lightning.

A SNOWMOBILE ACCIDENT

One cold winter evening I was called to take care of a man who was injured in a snowmobile accident. It was a crisp, cold, clear moonlit night. A group of snowmobilers were cruising on a farmer's snow-covered field north of Blair. One of the snowmobiles plunged over a cliff at the edge of the field. This cliff was unrecognizable as such in the deep snow. The snowmobile landed on the leg of the driver. When I saw this gentleman in the emergency room, he had multiple injuries to that leg. I immediately sent him to a trauma center in Omaha where a team of surgeons worked all night to try to save his leg. Unfortunately, they were unsuccessful.

MOTORCYCLES

I told all four of our children that if they even mentioned the word motorcycle to me, that "THEY WERE IN DEEP TROUBLE." Here are some of my many stories that illustrate the reason why I said that, and the benefit that came from that comment. Our daughter Kathleen, as a high school senior, turned down an offer to ride on a male classmate's new motorcycle. Her exact (exaggerated) words were, "If my dad found out, he would kill me." Another girl accepted the offer. After going only two or three blocks, they had an accident and the other girl sustained a broken femur (upper leg bone). It took the next six months for that broken leg to heal. Her mother and I were so proud of our daughter for refusing that ride.

Here is another tragic motorcycle story: Dr. Rath and I jointly examined a gentleman in his 50s who lived in mid-Nebraska, about one hundred miles from Blair. He had always wanted to own a Harley, so he and two of his sons came to Omaha to buy one. The father did not want to ride it in Omaha traffic, so one of the sons rode it to Blair, where his father took over. As he rounded a curve a mile or so north of Blair, he sideswiped an oncoming car. He lost his left leg because of that accident.

There used to be a motocross dirt-bike course on a farm located about ten or twelve miles north of Blair. They raced every Saturday, except in the winter. Almost every Saturday afternoon a major injury occurred there, keeping our emergency room busy. Thankfully, after a few years that race track was abandoned, and those racing injuries went away. Those of us who staffed the emergency room breathed a sigh of relief on Saturdays.

Carole and I were returning from a Nebraska-Missouri football game in Columbia, Missouri. We were driving on a two-lane highway in northwestern Missouri. I was driving the posted speed limit when a motorcycle passed me like I was standing still. Only a couple of minutes later I saw in the distance ahead a cloud of dust and a flash of a single headlight pointing skyward. When I arrived at the scene another carload of people had already stopped to help and had already called for a rescue squad. About all I could do was to direct cars to prevent them from running over the badly injured motorcyclist. As he was being loaded into the ambulance his survival appeared questionable.

What had happened was this—as the motorcyclist was passing a pickup that was pulling a horse trailer, the pickup turned left into a farm lane. The motorcyclist hit the horse trailer almost broadside. We read in the newspaper the next day that the motorcyclist had died.

A classmate of mine in medical school became a kidney transplant surgeon, who worked primarily in the major hospitals in Minneapolis, Minnesota. He was back in Omaha for a medical school class reunion the same year that the Nebraska State Legislature was first debating the law that requires all motorcyclists to wear a helmet. He commented to me, "If you guys pass that law, there goes the source of some of my kidneys." I passed that comment along to our local state legislator at the time. The state legislator thought a minute and replied, "Ya' know—I never looked at it that way before."

AN ACCIDENT-PRONE FAMILY

I cared for several large families whose children seemed to be accident-prone. Here is a story involving one such family. One night after a high school basketball game, several siblings from this family piled into the older brother's car. They had not gone very far when the car got hit by a train, and I was called to the scene by the first responders—our local rescue squad. Fortunately, there were no serious injuries; however one of the younger brothers in the back seat kept crying out, "Help, I have a broken leg." The rescue squad personnel were very quick to investigate. Sure enough, lying in the back seat, the young boy was pointing at the cast that I had placed on his leg several days previously for a break in that leg. Apparently, the kid was having his fun. His older brother, the driver of the car, was dinged on the head and it took him a few weeks to work out the bugs from his concussion. The younger brother, the one who already had the cast, had originally broken his leg when he was trying to hurdle a divided barn door and he did not make it. A year or two later, a teenage daughter from that same family got squeezed between a farm wagon and a farm building. The result was a tear in her liver. Dr. Rath and I had to operate to repair the tear and stop the bleeding. Everyone in that family was reported to be doing well as of 2016.

A VERY RARE EVENT

During the very early years of my practice in Blair, I was awakened by an urgent call from the hospital ER nurse, "Come quickly—we need you right now!" The rescue squad had arrived with a four-year-old boy who was not responding. Sadly, he already had no vital signs and nothing could be done. I had to confirm that he was dead on arrival.

Mom and Dad were frantic, as were we all. The boy had not been sick. He had gone to bed as usual. In the early morning he called out to his mother, "I am thirsty." He got up, wobbled a bit—and fell over dead.

We needed answers, so I picked up the telephone and called Dr. Rudy Schenken. He was the chief pathologist at Nebraska Methodist Hospital in Omaha where I had trained. Dr. Schenken was one of the most respected pathologists in the nation. He said, "Send him down and we will see what we can find." The boy's mom and dad agreed that a postmortem exam just had to be done, if for no other reason than to be sure that no guilty feelings would haunt them for the rest of their lives.

A few days later, the report was very surprising. The cause of death was rupture of the aorta, caused by invasion of the aortic arch by cancerous cells. The source of those cancerous cells was a persistent thyroglossal duct. One has to go back to the embryology textbook from medical school days, to understand this problem. The thyroglossal duct has its origin in the embryo seven or eight weeks after conception. Then a bud develops from the tissue which will eventually form the tongue, the thyroid gland, the hyoid bone, and adjacent structures. The thyroglossal duct normally disappears after these structures develop. Occasionally however, the duct or a small cyst near the thyroid gland will persist into adulthood. It is very rare for these cells to become malignant. However, in this case they did just that. The malignant cells eventually invaded the nearby aortic arch without any hint that anything was wrong, until disaster struck when the aorta ruptured, killing him instantly. I recently asked the boy's father if it was OK to include this story in this book. He agreed, but I could tell that the agony is still there after all of these many years—for all of us concerned.

MYASTHENIA GRAVIS
ANOTHER EXTREMELY RARE ILLNESS

Although myasthenia gravis is rare, I have witnessed two cases in my lifetime. There is no cure, but medication helps control the symptoms. The first person was an elderly man whom I saw in my office in the 1970s because he was having episodes during which he could not chew or swallow very well. It seemed as though his mouth and chewing could not coordinate themselves. He could not control his saliva and it kept dripping off of his chin. His speech became somewhat slurred. There seemed to be no paralysis. These episodes usually occurred when he was tired or not rested. A consultation with a neurologist yielded the diagnosis of myasthenia gravis. He was treated with a medicine which stimulated the production of a chemical which causes the brain to increase its production of a chemical called acetylcholine. This is a chemical involved in the stimulation of the nerves which initiate muscle contraction. His symptoms seemed much better while on that medicine.

The second case was not my patient, as the illness surfaced several years after I had retired. He and his wife were our good friends from our church.

I became involved when Carole and I went to visit him after he had been hospitalized with a suspected stroke. The patient's wife was not satisfied with the presumptive diagnosis of a "stroke." As a family friend, she asked me for my opinion. Although he was very confused, was very weak and could not stand by himself, there was no obvious paralysis. I tended to agree with his wife. She and the attending physician then arranged for consultation with a neurologist. That consultation produced the diagnosis of myasthenia gravis in crisis.

In more recent years, the medical profession had learned that myasthenia gravis is an autoimmune disease in which our own immune systems do not work very well as we age. There is no cure, but the symptoms of myasthenia gravis are now better controlled by periodic IV infusions of a blood product which is derived from donated blood. In turn, this blood is highly fractionated and pooled in the laboratory to produce hyper immune globulin. It is very expensive due to the processes involved to refine it. This friend of ours did very well with the periodic IV infusions until he passed away two or three years later. He was cared for mainly at the Veterans Hospital in Omaha as an outpatient during his last few years. He passed away of complications of this disease, but he did have a few good years because of the hyper-immune globulin infusions.

In the early years I treated a very obese gentleman for pancreatic cancer. His Omaha oncologist ordered weekly IV infusions of a cancer medicine called 5-Fluorouracil. We alternated weekly between his office and my office, thereby saving him many trips to Omaha. We managed to control his pain, although he lost a hundred pounds in the process. One day this patient jokingly said to me, "Ya know, Doc, if I had not been so fat when we started all of this, I would never have lasted this long, would I?" I had to agree, and we both chuckled. He passed away peacefully a short time after that conversation.

JURY DUTY

One of the responsibilities of U.S. citizenship is jury duty. Every physician dreads the call to jury duty, not because of any lack of respect for our civic responsibilities, but because it is impossible to make yourself available for jury duty on short notice, and still honor your obligations to your patients at the same time. My own experience is a good illustration of that point.

During the month of January in the early 1990s, I was called to jury duty for the U.S. Federal District Court in Omaha, Nebraska. I was to be available for the entire month during the height of the flu and pneumonia season. This is traditionally one of the busiest times of the year in a rural family practice setting. I was not thrilled, to say the least.

I reported to the U.S. Federal District Court in Omaha, some 25 miles to the south of Blair, at the appointed time. After standard instructions were given, I was selected for a potential jury panel in a case in which our own county sheriff was being sued for alleged abuse of a prisoner in our county jail. The usual presiding U.S. Federal judge was unavailable at that time, so a replacement from Kansas City was brought in. This judge turned out to be the brother of a prominent

Blair businessman, whose family I knew personally and professionally. Of course, the first question asked of each potential juror was, "Are you acquainted with the defendant?" My answer was, "Yes, he is my patient, and I have taken care of his heart and blood pressure problems for a number of years." The next question involved any knowledge of several other people who had been involved in the case. One person they mentioned was "Ray Kastanek"—the lawyer pronounced his name 'Kas-ta-NECK'—our local trooper from the Nebraska State Patrol. I raised my hand again and said, "Your Honor, his name is pronounced Ka-STAN-ek, and his wife, Sally, is one of my employees." At that point, the judge slowly took off his glasses and said, "Dr. Bagby, why don't you just go home. Nobody wants you on this jury."

The next day I returned to my busy office schedule, knowing that my availability for the rest of the month was on a day-to-day basis. One of the appointments that day was a long-time patient of mine. He had developed a hernia which he wished to have surgically repaired during the next week. This patient knew that standard procedure at our local hospital was for me, the referring physician, to serve as first assistant to our surgeon during the procedure.

After I explained to him that although there was no problem scheduling the procedure, he was very disappointed to learn that there was the possibility that I would not be there. He thought about it for a few moments, then said as he was walking out of the office, "I'll see what I can do." I was puzzled, as I did not know what he meant until I received a telephone call the next morning. It was the clerk of the Federal District Court in Omaha, who said, "Dr. Bagby, my BROTHER visited with me last evening. Why don't you just take care of my brother's problem and forget all about showing up down here anymore. We can do just fine without you." Thus ended my jury duty obligation. The surgery was accomplished with no problems. This story eventually ended up on the bulletin board in the lawyer's lounge at the Douglas County Courthouse, courtesy of my good lifelong friend, Omaha lawyer Roger Holthaus.

CONSTIPATION IN THE ELDERLY, CAUSED BY A PARATHYROID ADENOMA

One of the frequent challenges in caring for elderly patients is treating constipation. Usually the problem is due to decreased fluid and fiber intake. We must also consider colon cancer. This particular elderly lady, who lived in a nursing home, remained constipated in spite of all the usual tests and interventions.

A lab test revealed a very high serum calcium level, which led me to suspect hyperparathyroidism. The next lab test revealed a very high blood level of the hormone that is produced by the parathyroid glands. I consulted with our radiologist, Dr. Howard Hunt. He advised me which x-rays to order to demonstrate what we suspected, the presence of a large parathyroid adenoma. The enlarged gland was producing too much parathyroid hormone, which was the reason for the constipation. It had to be benign, because cancer cells would not be producing the hormone at all.

This was before the advent of ultrasound imaging. Had that been available then, our search would have been much easier. Everyone has a total of four tiny parathyroid glands which are tucked in between the back side of the thyroid gland and next to the trachea. They regulate the calcium level in the blood. Not enough calcium can cause muscle spasms, and too much calcium causes muscles to become weak. As long as at least one of the four parathyroid glands is intact and functioning well, everything is OK. And so, after Dr. Hunt established which one of the four parathyroid glands in the neck was the offender, I referred the patient to a very good neck surgeon in Omaha. This surgeon had trained for this very operation at the prestigious M.D. Anderson Hospital in Houston, Texas. After the very delicate, successful surgery, he called to congratulate Dr. Hunt and me for making the correct diagnosis of this rare and unusual condition.

THE VALUE OF SURROUNDING YOURSELF WITH GOOD PEOPLE

I JOINED THE Blair Clinic in 1964. I had spent a couple of years in the U.S. Army in a dispensary setting, not really being able to take care of anyone who was sick. So, after discharge from the Army, I took some further training in surgery and obstetrics at Nebraska Methodist Hospital in Omaha.

While there I discovered that the Blair doctors were desperate to recruit a new doctor. Dr. Rudy Sievers was the Nebraska State Medical Association president that year (1964). The obligations of that office required him to be out of town frequently. Since Dr. Howard was semi-retired, Dr. Leslie Grace was very overworked. It was a great opportunity to become associated with a fine group of doctors who had the respect of the entire Nebraska State Medical Association. I joined them and I was welcomed by everyone.

As the years went by at the Blair Clinic, we all became busier, and several other doctors came for varying lengths of time, then left for various reasons. In the late 1960s, during the creation of a three-year Family Practice residency program at the Medical School in Omaha, Dr. Sievers was asked if he would assume the chairmanship of that program. He told us that he refused because he just could not bear the thought of leaving the three of us with such a heavy load of patients to look after at the Blair Clinic. It was a wonderful opportunity for him, but we were grateful that he refused to leave.

Given our situation, it felt like we hit the jackpot when Dr. Richard Gentry joined us. The following is his story.

Dr. Richard Gentry

Dick's parents, Max and Emily Gentry, were Nebraska Wesleyan graduates in the 1920s. Max went on to earn his M.D. He ran a mission hospital in Chunking (Chongqing), China, where Dick was born in 1930. After the Japanese began open warfare against China in 1937, the family was forced to leave in the late 1930s. They settled in Gering, Nebraska. All four of the children were boys; Dick was the youngest. His mother, Emily, was named the Nebraska Mother of the Year in the 1950s.

When I was a freshman at Nebraska Wesleyan University in 1952, Dick had just left Wesleyan to start medical school that year, but the legends of his academic achievements are still well known there. His future wife, Marilyn Hunkins, was still a senior at Wesleyan that year, and I met her when we were both members of the Wesleyan Concert Band, where she played French horn. She told me a lot about Dick, including that, like me, he also played the clarinet.

Dick was drafted into the U.S. Army about the same time as I, during the military buildup after the Berlin Wall went up. He was in his second year as a surgical resident at Sacramento General Hospital in California. He spent his military time at a surgical hospital in Virginia, while I served in the medical corps at Fort Knox and then in Korea. After discharge, Dick settled in Falls City, Nebraska, and I settled in Blair. I got to know Dick better through the Nebraska State Medical Association.

One day in the winter of 1976-77, when all of us at the Blair Clinic were busier than a one-armed paper hanger, I received a telephone call from Dick. I shall never forget that conversation. Dick said, "Chuck, you may think that this is a strange phone call, but there has to be a better place to live than Falls City, Nebraska." I almost fainted. After I regained my composure, I asked Dick to tell me the story. Dick was prompted to leave a thriving, busy practice in Falls City for one reason. That town would not support its school system.

Education was important to Dick and his family. After all, Dick's father was an M.D., Dick and two older brothers were M.D.s, and another older brother was a Ph.D. chemist. Dick may have been one of the few doctors I have ever known who graduated first in his class in grade school, high school, college and medical school. Education was high on his list of priorities. Anyway, Dick had been on the Falls City school board for several years. The citizens of the town had just rejected a school bond issue, for the second time around. This time they even elected some new school board members who then proceeded to sell the land that the previous school board had acquired with the intentions of building a new high school. Dick and his partner looked at each other and said, "Well, if they do not want to educate our children, we will just move somewhere where they do."

When Dick visited Blair to have a closer look at our town, he did not even visit our clinic or the hospital; he already knew what he needed to know about us from the medical standpoint. I made appointments for him to visit with two people while he was here—Gordon Patterson, the pastor of the Methodist Church, and Jerry Otte, the high school principal. Jerry later became the Blair superintendent of schools.

Within less than six months from that initial phone call, both Dr. Gentry and his partner in Falls City pulled up stakes and left town. Dick, his wife Marilyn, and their high school freshman daughter, Carol, moved to Blair. Their three older children were already in college or professional school. That move took conviction, courage, and immediately reinforced my admiration. Dick's retired in-laws, Mildred and Lyle Hunkins, later moved to Blair.

Blair was very fortunate and grateful for the presence of the Gentry family. Dick and Marilyn were stellar citizens and community leaders of Blair. They were active in the Methodist Church, and both were in the choirs and in numerous other leadership roles. He was a skilled mediator and he was able to smooth out ruffled feathers when the need arose. Dick and his father-in-law were long time Lions Club members. Their youngest daughter, Carol, attended and graduated from Blair High School and played in the Band and on the volleyball team. Dick and Marilyn were avid bridge club competitors.

Dick was unquestionably the backbone of the Blair medical community from the late 1970s until his untimely death from prostate cancer in 1997, at the age of 64. The medical community and everyone in Blair was devastated by his passing.

Dick was diagnosed with a very aggressive prostate cancer in the late 1980s. The PSA blood test level was zero. The pathologist theorized that the cancer cells were so undifferentiated that they were unable to produce any prostate specific antigen at all. Dick received the entire spectrum of available treatments, including a trip to M.D. Anderson Hospital in Houston for their evaluations. Dick soldiered on for eight years, still seeing his patients, who were eager to see him. One of those patients was my wife's mother. Like many patients, she asked Dick, as he came into the examining room, "How are you doing?" His answer was, "More to the point, how are you doing?" That answer skillfully deflected the attention away from him and back to the patient.

One day, after viewing a ghastly-looking recent chest x-ray, I went back to the office and sat down beside him and said, "Dick, why don't you just take off and do anything that you ever wanted to do?" He put his hand on my shoulder and said, "Chuck, I *am* doing what I always wanted to do." We lowered the American flag at the Blair Hospital to half-staff on Labor Day, 1997, the day he passed away—20 years to the day after he moved to Blair.

I had the opportunity recently to talk with a banker from Falls City. Of course he already knew Dick Gentry's story. He told me that it took twenty years for the community of Falls City to recover from the loss of two of their five doctors so suddenly. After twenty years Falls City finally got their new school, and were able to introduce computer science into the curriculum. Dick told me that the reason those two bond issues had failed was that most of the opposition were retired farmers who had already educated their own children, and were opposed to paying further taxes to educate the kids of their friends and neighbors, and the families of those who take care of you—like your doctors, dentists, lawyers, etc., etc. The lesson here is that if you want good people to move to and live in your town, then you must be willing to give their children a quality education.

Dr. HOWARD HUNT

Dr. Hunt was a physician whom I shall always remember as a great mentor in every phase of medicine. He was a nationally-recognized radiologist who brought the first cobalt radiation unit to Nebraska at Omaha's Methodist Hospital in the late 1940s. He successfully treated the largest number of cases of cervical cancer in the nation with cobalt radiation. To document the cases, he created a cancer registry at the Methodist Hospital. For this he received a gold medal from the American College of Radiology. He was a graduate of Harvard University medical school and trained in radiology at the University of Michigan. He was the chief of radiology during my internship at the Methodist Hospital in 1960-61. He also was chief of the department of radiology at the University of Nebraska College of Medicine.

One day, when I was an intern, I was rounding with Dr. Hunt when he noticed a large brownish-colored seborrheic keratosis, a benign mole, on the face of one of his patients. With the patient's permission, he proceeded to show me a great method to remove such a lesion. He called for a nurse to bring him the needed equipment. Right there in the patient's bed, he swabbed the lesion with alcohol, infiltrated under it with local anesthetic, removed the lesion with electrocautery and surgical curettage down to, but not through the dermis layer of skin. Then he lightly controlled the bloody ooze with the electrocautery. He assured me and the patient that the scab would fall off nicely in 10 days to two weeks, with absolutely no scar. I used this technique many times for the 40-plus years of my practice. Fast, easy and at minimal cost. All this from a nationally recognized radiologist and radiotherapist. This was not even his specialty.

Besides being the head of radiology at Methodist Hospital, he soon became chief of radiology at the University of Nebraska College of Medicine in Omaha. That was his status when I arrived on the scene in Blair in 1964.

Dr. George Pullman was the radiologist in Blair when I arrived in 1964. A couple of years later, Dr. Pullman decided to retire. We were at a loss as to whom we could recruit to replace him. Since I had trained with Dr. Hunt and knew him well, I offered to go to Omaha, and ask Dr. Hunt if he knew of anyone who might be currently available. He thought for a few minutes, and then he said, "I am about to retire—(in the 1960s, the university had a hard and fast rule that all department heads had to retire at age 65)—why don't I just drive to Blair three days a week and do all of your diagnostic radiology for you?" After that happened, doctors from all over the state, from Scottsbluff and Alliance to Falls City, asked me, "How in the world did you accomplish that?" Boy, were they envious. After he came to Blair, I would hear an occasional comment from a patient mentioning that they were uncomfortable about having Floyd Hinz, our long-time hospital maintenance engineer, take their x-rays. Dr. Hunt could recognize talent when he saw it. He had personally taught Floyd the art of taking good x-rays, starting with the basics of radiology which includes not only correct exposure, but equally importantly, correct anatomic positioning. Those patients became more accepting when they learned that Floyd had been personally trained by Dr. Hunt himself. I learned so much medicine from Dr. Hunt. He would not only show me what he was seeing on the x-rays—then he would proceed to suggest the best treatment for the patient. And he almost always was correct.

One time I was showing him an x-ray of an elderly, hospitalized nursing home patient who had a pathologic fracture of her femur (upper leg bone). The bone just broke while the patient was turning over in bed. Radiation can cause long term weakening of bone and increase the chances of a fracture, sometimes years later. That is exactly what happened in this instance. Dr. Hunt glanced at the name on the film and exclaimed, "I know her, I treated her years ago with cobalt radiation for cancer of the cervix." He jumped up, and down the hall he went to her hospital room and together they threw their arms around each other.

I recall this particular story about Dr. Hunt. Our Blair hospital (Memorial Community Hospital was the official name in those days) was being surveyed by the Joint Commission for the Accreditation of Hospitals. This was a required periodic survey by this national certifying agency. The survey is so detailed and picky that it gets everyone's attention. I was chief of the medical staff on that occasion, which is how I heard this story directly from the surveyor. The surveyor was in the radiology department grilling Dr. Hunt, who became very upset with him. The surveyor told me, "This little old man jumped up onto the x-ray table saying loudly, "Don't YOU try to tell ME how to run an x-ray department!" After they checked his credentials, we passed with flying colors. Dr. Hunt continued to serve as our resident radiologist for the next 17 years, until he was 82 years old.

Dr. HANS RATH

Dr. Hans Rath was an invaluable general surgeon who served us wonderfully for many years. His parents were of German heritage, part of the Germans who immigrated to Russia in the late 1700s at the invitation of Catherine the Great. At the time of the Russian revolution, the entire family was able to escape to the United States, where they settled in Nebraska.

His patients usually did well because he handled their tissues very gently during the operation. The nurses always gave him the royal treatment. I always felt comfortable assisting him with any operation. He traveled from his home in Omaha almost on a daily basis. He was also on the staff at Nebraska Methodist and at Bishop Clarkson Hospitals in Omaha, and many rural hospitals in the area. I have already mentioned him in connection with several patients in this book.

Here is another. One Sunday evening when I was on call at our Blair hospital emergency room, we operated upon three patients, each with an acutely infected appendix, and a fourth patient with an incarcerated femoral hernia. All four of these patients required prompt surgery.

About five p.m. I had called Dr. Rath to come to Blair to perform an appendectomy. During the thirty minutes that it took him to arrive, another patient with right lower-quadrant abdominal pain presented to the emergency room. This patient also had appendicitis. While we were in the operating room with the second appendicitis patient, here came a third. And before we finished taking care of the third case of appendicitis, a lady with an incarcerated femoral hernia was admitted to the ER. I am sure that you already know that a case of appendicitis needs to be taken care of promptly before it ruptures. Likewise, an incarcerated femoral hernia should be taken to surgery promptly before the contents of the hernia sac–usually bowel–swells so much as to cut off its own blood supply. Six p.m. to seven a.m. the next morning was a long and busy night for all of us.

While preparing for an operation (while scrubbing my hands and donning my sterile garb) I often prayed for guidance and steady hands. A bit of humor in the midst of an arduous and difficult operation does help ease the tension and help lighten the atmosphere. One day I helped Dr. Rath with a particularly long and bloodier operation than usual. I will spare you the details, except for this: halfway through the operation, my scrub pants became untied and dropped to the floor (whoops!). Since I already was wearing a long surgical gown over them I just stepped out of the pants, and the operation went on uninterrupted.

After the procedure was finished the cleanup crew took over. As they were working hard, one of the cleaning ladies presented herself at the operating room door. She held up my bloodied pair of scrub pants, and loudly announced, "This room is a mess! But what I really want to know is, whose pants are these?" The cleanup crew would remind me of that incident for many years afterwards.

Speaking of humor in the operating room, Dr. Rath always enjoyed a good pun. He was about four inches shorter than I. Every time that I was his first assistant in the operating room he would ask for his "growth hormone"—a four-inch-high platform on which he stood. That way our arms and hands would be working at the same level.

The final step of preparation before the start of most any operation is to isolate the operative field with a long head-to-toe sterile drape with a cutout directly over the appropriate spot. Dr. Rath would align that cutout over the operative field. He then took one end of the folded sterile drape and placed it over the foot of the operating table, saying, "To de feet." Then, as he spread the other end of the sterile drape above the patient's head (creating a protected work area for the anesthetists), Dr. Rath dutifully recited, "and here's to Victory."

Another pun or joke that he repeated at almost every operation requires a bit of explanation. It is standard operating procedure for the charge nurse, before the start every surgical procedure to ask, "Doctor, what is your pre-operative diagnosis?" The answer is then duly recorded in the record. At the end of the operation, this question is then modified to, "Doctor, what is your post-operative diagnosis?"

Dr. Rath's usual answer to that question was, "Sam Ting."

The explanation goes like this. One day an American tourist and his wife were strolling along the street in San Francisco's Chinatown. Their curiosity was aroused when they saw a sign on an establishment that read, "Ole Olsen's Chinese Laundry." So, they entered the establishment and asked to see the owner. This small Chinese man came out to greet them. He said, "Yes, my name is Ole Olsen." The American couple asked him how he came to acquire that name. His answer was this: "When I immigrated to the United States, I was standing in the registration line. They asked the man in front of me, 'What is your name?' His name was Ole Olsen. So, when it was my turn I replied to that question 'Sam Ting.' And I have been known as Ole Olsen ever since." And so, Dr. Rath's post-operative diagnosis was usually, "Sam Ting."

At the conclusion of another operation, as is sometimes the case, the patient was a bit slow to wake up, even though his vital signs were normal. Dr. Rath walked over and in a loud voice said to the patient, "LAZARUS, wake up!" And he did.

I shall always feel indebted to Dr. Rath for his nomination of me, as an alumnus of the Nebraska College of Medicine, to become a member of Alpha Omega Alpha. AΩA is the honor society whose members encompass the entire medical profession. A medical student can be considered for induction to AΩA if they place in the top 10% academically of their junior or senior class. In 2005 I was elected to membership as an alumnus because of my work mentoring medical students during their rural preceptorship program. The motto of this organization is "Be Worthy to Serve the Suffering." I was very humbled to become a member of that organization, alongside my colleagues Drs. Sievers, Grace, Gentry, Howard Hunt, Hans Rath, and many other mentors along this journey.

AN ENCOUNTER WITH JIMSONWEED POISONING

IT IS UNUSUAL for a family doctor to encounter a case of human poisoning by jimsonweed. It is more common for this problem to be seen in livestock. It was reported that the early settlers had been affected by jimsonweed poisoning near Jamestown, Virginia, in the 1600s. It is called by various names, such as loco weed. The weeds produce a neurotoxin called "swainsonine." This chemical has an effect like an overdose of atropine—very fast heart rate, very high fevers, hallucinations, extremely dry mouth and neurotoxicity, even death. I encountered my one and only case in the wee hours one morning when the Blair police brought in a young man to our local hospital's emergency room. The police had been called because a small group of young people were creating a disturbance wandering in the middle of Washington street, at the 19th Street intersection near the west edge of downtown Blair. They thought that they were leprechauns, and they were running and shouting all over the place. They were harassing people in their cars at that intersection.

The one that I was asked to see was not only hallucinating, he was also very sick. He had a dry tongue, a fever of over 104 degrees F., and a tachycardia (fast heart rate) of 160 to 200 beats/minute. These symptoms and findings were very suggestive of atropine overdose. One of his fellow "leprechauns" who was not so sick, mentioned that they had been sampling some flowering plants that had been planted along the curb at a house located a few blocks away. These plants were later identified as jimsonweed. The local police dealt with that issue. Since the young man's blood pressure was OK and he was breathing OK, and was not in congestive heart failure, I filled him full of IV fluids, got his temp down with ice packs, etc. until we flushed the poison out of his system via his kidneys. In a couple of days he had recovered. Note: It is probably better NOT to encounter leprechauns in this fashion.

COURAGE: "SOLDIER ON"

I USED TO tell patients with a chronic or a fatal diagnosis to "hang in there." However, I think I like the phrase "Soldier On" better. There are memories of my years in practice that are very heart-warming. I fondly remember a number of patients whose inner courage rose to the surface when they or their families were faced with illness, disability, or even certain death.

One such lady, in her early 60s, lived alone in a small home near Herman—a small town some ten miles to the north of Blair. She was so severely disabled with advanced rheumatoid arthritis that she could barely walk. She so looked forward to reaching Medicare eligibility so that she could get one of those new-fangled hip replacements. She had such deformity of her hands and fingers that she could barely hold anything. She also had COPD, a chronic lung problem which required the use of an inhaler. However, she did not have the strength in her hands or fingers to actuate the inhaler. The hospital respiratory therapist helped with the problem by building a collection chamber to attach to the inhaler. Then she could place the inhaler on a table, steady it against one hand, and press on the top of the inhaler with a closed fist of the other hand. The mist would be retained in the chamber attached to the inhaler until she could get the chamber to her mouth to inhale.

This chamber device became commercially available a few years later. Her third significant problem was that she was totally blind, the result of failed bilateral corneal transplants. She was able to live alone with housekeeping help, only because she had memorized the exact location of every single object inside her home. Everything always had to be in the exact same place. What a courageous lady she was! She was so very appreciative of anything that we could do for her. Sadly, as I remember, she did not live long enough to have her hip replaced.

One family that I shall always remember were patients for almost the entire duration of my active practice in Blair. Their children and our children were classmates all through their school years. One of their boys was a very good athlete in all sports at a young age. His father brought him into the office to find the cause a sore back when he was a freshman in high school. X-rays revealed a major bony defect in his back that required a spinal fusion. He sat out all athletics his sophomore year in a body cast. The spinal fusion was successful and healed well enough to allow him to play basketball during his junior year. By the time he was a senior, he was named to our local high school all-conference teams in both basketball and football. Tom Osborne had invited him to walk on at Nebraska to try for a football scholarship. He opted, instead, for an academic college scholarship elsewhere. He eventually became a successful physical therapist.

His father was a former athlete who, a number of years ago, had some unresolving lower abdominal discomfort for several days before seeking medical attention. Over the years, I have noticed that athletes tend to delay medical attention when prompt medical attention would have created a better outcome. (I still have a weak left ankle myself as proof of that statement.) When he did come to see me, he had a ruptured appendix with a large abscess. Postoperative he was given a lot of appropriate antibiotics. Over the next several years, he had adhesion problems with his bowel related to that ruptured appendix. The first time that the adhesions obstructed him, surgery was required to release the blockage. But after that we could pass a long tube by mouth which would end up in the small bowel, thus relieving the obstruction. He would be symptom-free between these bouts, which became progressively less severe and further apart as the years passed by. He had been feeling fine, with no abdominal symptoms for about a year or more.

Then one day shortly after Thanksgiving, he came to my office asking for a general checkup. He had no specific symptoms or complaints, and my review of systems and physical findings turned up nothing. And yet, I sensed that something must be going on because, as we talked he kept mentioning his wife and his love and concern for her.

As he left the office, I still had that uneasy feeling, because something seemed different about him. A couple of weeks later we got our answer. He had been hanging up Christmas lights at his home. He fell off of the ladder—striking his head as he fell. Subsequent head X-rays and scans revealed a frontal lobe brain tumor. He was referred to a very good neurosurgeon in Omaha. The tumor was judged to be inoperable. The neurosurgeon had to give him the devastating news that he had about six months to live.

This news came just before Christmas. This was a huge blow to their entire family, and to me, and to the entire community of Blair. The next six months were hard, extremely hard, but "Soldier On" they did. One Sunday morning almost exactly six months later, I received a phone call at church from his wife, asking me to come to their home right away. When I arrived, his wife was holding her lifeless husband close to her heart. I cried right along with her for a while until I finally picked up the telephone to call the mortician for her.

His wife had held a part-time position working for our hospital in Blair for many years. She continued in that capacity after her husband's death. About a year or so later, she stopped me in the hospital hallway to ask my opinion. She was considering taking flight training so that she could obtain a pilot's license and then fly her own airplane. I told her that I was proud of her gumption, and to "go for it." She did. This is what I mean by "Soldiering On."

Another young man, with a young family, had a terminal brain cancer. His young wife had to continue working to pay the bills. She had a very good job. His parents lived in a small home in a nearby town. His parents put a bed in their living room and took care of him and the children during the day while his wife continued to work. His wife did manage to be in church every Sunday during his illness; the support that our church gave the family was wonderful also. It was heart-warming to see that kind of family devotion.

Another case I remember is that of a gentleman who was a local farmer. He had been run over by his own tractor.

I met him at the emergency room door, helping to unload him from the ambulance. The most serious of his many injuries was a shattered right hip joint. The femoral head and neck and the acetabulum were all crushed like an egg shell. After all of this crushed bone fused together into one solid mass, and all of his other injuries, including another fracture lower down on the same leg, healed, he then received a new total hip replacement. This was in the 1970s, when total hip replacement was a very new surgical procedure. Having never seen that operation before, I went down to Clarkson Hospital in Omaha to observe the surgery. He still walks with a decided limp after 30+ years.

One day I fielded a call outside of office hours. This young couple had recently arrived home from vacation. The husband had suddenly developed difficulty with the vision in one eye. On exam, I noticed that the muscles that control the movement of that eye were malfunctioning. Something was wrong with the oculomotor nerve in the brain. I sent him to a neurosurgeon for an evaluation. We were all surprised when the report was that the nerve had been invaded by a metastatic cancer, the origin of which proved to be a lung cancer. There had been no pulmonary symptoms. His widow still is involved in a business here in Blair, and I say a silent little prayer for both of them whenever I see her.

Another young lady, with four children, lost her 30-some-year-old husband to a right-sided colon cancer. In this location, cancers of the colon are often silent for a long time before offering symptoms. However, it is unusual to encounter this problem in this age group. His widow and his children still do a commendable job of soldiering on.

THE EVOLUTION OF RESCUE SQUADS

The mortician's hearse to the use of helicopters

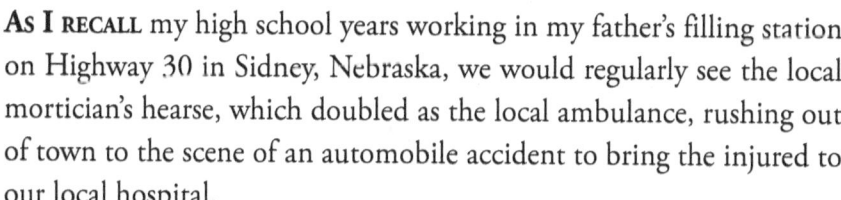

As I recall my high school years working in my father's filling station on Highway 30 in Sidney, Nebraska, we would regularly see the local mortician's hearse, which doubled as the local ambulance, rushing out of town to the scene of an automobile accident to bring the injured to our local hospital.

I have mentioned, earlier in this book, about my service in the U.S. Army. Here is the full story of what happened.

I finished my internship in June of 1961. The Korean conflict was ten years behind us. We knew that there had been no doctors drafted during that span of years. Therefore, almost all of my group of interns made plans not involving the military. We had been planning for several months to join my wife's older brother in a general practice in Greeley, Colorado. I had applied for a Colorado license; we purchased a home in Greeley, and were just starting to get established.

Then, in August 1961, just two months later, the East Germans built the Berlin Wall, a major event in the Cold War. For most of my intern class, the Berlin Wall changed everything. Within four months I was drafted as a captain in the Medical Corps of the United States Army. My draft notice arrived in the mail on the day after Thanksgiving.

My induction was delayed until after our second son, Richard, was born in Greeley on Dec. 10, 1961. A few days later Carole's mother was arriving on the Union Pacific Streamliner to stay until after Christmas to help with our new son. I was waiting at the train station. The streamliner seemed to be running late. I inquired at the depot and was informed that it had hit a truck a couple of miles out of town. I decided to investigate and I found that it was not a truck, but rather a fully loaded school bus that was hit. All twenty children in the back of the bus were killed instantly. I jumped out to help load survivors from the front of the bus into the available ambulances, which were arriving at about the same time as I did. They were mostly hearses which doubled as ambulances. I then went on to help at the hospital to help as I could in the emergency room. That was my horrific introduction to mass casualties and triage.

That was a real blow to that community, as well as to me personally. It was the featured story in LIFE magazine the next week.

When I began my practice in Blair in 1964, our local fire department had recently organized a rescue squad with local firemen as the first members. Their first ambulance was an older white panel delivery truck. Slowly but surely, the equipment and the training of the Emergency Medical Technicians (EMTs) improved in quality with each passing year. The impetus for all of this progress came from the experiences of returning veterans—from WWII, and especially the Korean War. This was particularly true of the increasing use of the helicopter as a means of rapid transport. One particular incident serves to point out the fact that the old and the new ways have to interact.

One blustery winter evening our local rescue squad brought in a long-time patient of mine, a retired local County Sheriff who had severe abdominal pain. It did not take long to diagnose a dissecting abdominal aortic aneurysm, confirmed by an across-the-table abdominal x-ray (a side view of the patient's abdomen while lying down on the x-ray table). The rescue squad personnel were still there doing the lifting on and off the x-ray table, and with a storm forecast to hit us within the hour, I had them load him right back up and drive directly to the closest trauma center, at Creighton University in Omaha.

The next morning the vascular surgeon called me to report a successful operation that saved the patient's life. Then he proceeded to chew me out for not sending the patient by helicopter. I calmly explained the circumstances - the impending storm, and the rescue squad personnel already there and chomping at the bit to get going. I pointed out that the trip to Omaha took less than 30 minutes, which meant the patient arrived at about the same time the helicopter would just have been landing in Blair - and as the storm had hit Blair by then, the helicopter might not have been able to take off again. It took the rescue squad more than two hours to return. The surgeon conceded the wisdom of my choice.

Reverend Harold Schaible, a local Blair pastor who later retired in Blair, was a combat medic in General Patton's army from North Africa all through Sicily, France and the Battle of the Bulge. As part of that journey he earned two purple hearts and a bronze star for valor. His wife told me the mortality rate among medics in Patton's army was 95%. He survived the war to become a pastor.

One of his early pastorates was in the eastern edge of the Nebraska Sandhills. These are the wide-open spaces of cattle country. He found that they had no local rescue squad. He became a pioneer in the movement to bring organized and trained rescue squads to the more sparsely populated areas of Nebraska. He took it upon himself to organize and train volunteers, including his young wife, and helped them obtain certification as emergency medical technicians (EMTs). He was later officially recognized by the appropriate state officials for his efforts. Today, it is so wonderful that the equipment and the training is outstanding. We really owe all of our rescue squad organizations a big thank you, especially the ones who are volunteers.

I have to tell one more story about this topic: For a few years, back in the late 1960s or 70s we had a physician in Blair who was a bit eccentric. He was partially deaf, having lost some of his hearing on the flight line at the Air Force base on Saipan, during WWII. He had served a few years as Nebraska's State Health Director under Governor Norbert Tiemann. As part of that job, he had acquired some experience in electronic communication. To his credit, he pushed the right buttons to get our local hospital, the rescue squad and the local police interconnected by radio. To demonstrate this to some of our hospital's nurses and me, he proceeded to pick up the transmitter and say "THIS IS A TEST—THIS IS A TEST— THIS IS A TEST." He then proceeded to describe a terrible airplane crash at the Blair Municipal Airport. He did not know that, besides the police and rescue squad members, there are a lot of private citizens in Blair who have police scanners. Several missed the message that this was a test. This caused quite a commotion around town that evening and the next morning!

UNUSUAL PRESENTATION OF PERNICIOUS ANEMIA AND TETANUS

I HAVE A couple pernicious anemia stories. One lady had a history of pernicious anemia, and a number of peripheral neuropathy (nerve damage) findings to go with it. She had numbness and tingling in her legs and her balance was not all that good. Her more than once-a-month shots of B12 helped those symptoms a lot. One day, she had some back pain symptoms, so she stopped to see a local chiropractor whose office was near where she lived. In the process of manipulating her back or neck, she suddenly could not move her legs at all. The chiropractor called the rescue squad, and then called me to ask if I would see her at the hospital. After I examined her in the ER, I gave her a shot of B12 and her symptoms rapidly improved. The chiropractor breathed easier after that.

Another pernicious anemia story involves a young adult man who was brought to the office one day by his family. He had to be helped in as he could barely walk. He seemed confused, his legs would hardly function, and he was pale. This illness seemed to have an acute onset. A stat blood count revealed a megaloblastic anemia—the textbook picture of pernicious anemia. We were able to get a vitamin B12 level on the blood sample, and that level was extremely low. Daily large doses of B12, given by shot, caused his symptoms to totally resolve in just a few days. He walked into the office the next week a totally symptom-free, normal man—amazing. This was the one case of PA that I saw from onset to resolution. A monthly B12 shot, for the rest of his life, should control the pernicious anemia.

TETANUS

I had another once in-a-lifetime case, this one involving tetanus. We all grow up understanding that if we get a cut or a deep scrape, particularly if it is contaminated such as stepping on a rusty nail, we should get a tetanus booster shot. Tetanus is included in the series of three immunizations that are routinely given to infants starting at age two months. But do any of you really know what tetanus does to you? The medical textbooks describe severe generalized muscle spasms which can even cause death by paralysis of the muscles used in breathing.

This patient was a middle-aged farmer near Craig, Nebraska. The Craig rescue squad brought him in one day after a heavy farm implement had fallen on his arm and shoulder. He had been harrowing his land preparing it for planting. One of the curved harrow blades had punctured his arm. There was little bleeding, and no fractures. He had been in the Army in the past, and I knew that the military is very religious about keeping the tetanus booster shots current. Therefore, with this injury we gave him another tetanus booster. I cleaned the wound as thoroughly as I could, and started him on antibiotics.

I let him go home, but two days later he presented with extremely painful muscle spasms in one leg, so severe that he would scream in pain. Any sort of stimulation, such as noise or touching any part of his body, would set off the spasms again. These were obvious tetanus type of muscle contractions, but limited to one extremity—and it was the leg on the opposite side of his body from the arm injury. This was not a textbook description of tetanus. There was one way to find out, and that was to administer tetanus antitoxin.

The only problem was that this patient was allergic to horse serum, and that involves how this particular antitoxin is produced—by using serum harvested from horses that had purposely been inoculated with the tetanus organism. Fortunately, human tetanus antitoxin had very recently been produced in a laboratory in Pennsylvania. We were able to get a supply flown to Omaha.

While we were waiting for the serum to arrive we took him to surgery. Dr. Rath opened and enlarged his wound and vigorously irrigated some deeply imbedded debris out of it. Interestingly, the long, curved harrow blade had penetrated deeply into the biceps muscle, burrowing most of eight to ten inches into the muscle under the skin, most probably depositing millions of tetanus organisms deep in the muscle. We had to lay open all of that tissue surgically in order to thoroughly clean out the wound. Within hours of administering human tetanus antitoxin to this suffering man, his symptoms vanished—never to return.

I did find one line in one medical journal that mentioned that there have been a few reported cases of tetanus spasms limited to one extremity, rather than involving the entire body as is the usual case. I also have no explanation as to why his previous immunizations and boosters did not protect him. I speculated that in spite of this, his immune system was simply overwhelmed by the massive inoculation of tetanus organisms by the harrow injury.

THE HOUSE WITH A RED LANTERN OVER THE DOOR

THIS UNNAMED LADY was one of my first patients. Soon after I joined the Blair Clinic in 1964, my senior partner asked me to take over the care of a ninety-some-year-old lady who was the only human occupant of a large two-story house located across the street from the old Blair passenger train depot (both the house and the depot were torn down many years ago). She shared the home with at least a dozen or more cats. I quickly learned that I had to be careful where I stepped—and even more careful where I sat. The lady of the house was nearly blind. On the wall were several pictures of a very attractive lady who was wearing the attire of the early 1900s. My senior partner told me that many years ago, there was a red lantern over the door.

This unfortunate lady had a colostomy that required medical attention every few weeks. During one of the worst winter blizzards that I can recall, she called the rescue squad to take her to the hospital. They had to use a snow plow to get her there. She had panicked with the thought that she might not get help if she needed it.

Dr. Rudy Sievers told me a story about an elderly couple in his office, back the 1940s or '50s. Somehow the conversation came around to that red lantern over the door of that house. The husband smiled, and his wife gave him a quick poke in the ribs. That ended that discussion.

ALCOHOL-RELATED STORIES

—∽∼—

FOR SEVERAL YEARS, the only occasions that I ever saw this lady (whom we shall call Marie) were when the local rescue squad delivered her to the hospital in an acute alcoholic stupor. Marie lived alone and her only source of income was her social security. She had a gentlemen friend, who joined her in her drinking binges on occasion, but (by his own admission) he was really only interested in sponging off her meager social security check.

Each episode was similar. She would present with extremely high blood alcohol levels and would be totally unconscious for two or three days. Treatment was supportive, consisting of fluid and electrolyte therapy, and medication if needed to keep her out of delirium tremens (extremely agitated confusion) as she progressed into her withdrawal period. After several days she would wake up enough so that we could have a coherent discussion. We worked on her nutrition and vitamin deficiencies, engaged social services to help at home, and we did everything that we could to help her stay dry. After a good drying out period she would return home only to return several months later with exactly the same problem.

After about the third or fourth admission for this same thing I was getting a bit frustrated. She woke up from her alcoholic stupor on the third day, and as I entered her hospital room that morning, I launched into a rather lengthy lecture about the evils of alcohol. She listened very attentively. When I was finished she looked me straight in the eye and very seriously stated, "I promise that I will be good, and I will never ever take another drink of alcohol." There was a moment of silence as we stared at each other, eye to eye. And then she said, "And if you believe that, I have this bridge that I would like to sell you."

We both had a good belly laugh over that remark. Marie never did change her ways, but we understood each other. When she would resume her binge drinking, I would do what I could for her. Eventually, alcohol won the battle.

The battle with alcoholic patients takes many different forms. During my middle years of practice, I was awakened about five a.m. one Sunday morning to take care of the driver of an automobile who was involved in an accident. This was a young man in his early 20s who had stolen a Pontiac Firebird in Sioux Falls, South Dakota, about 160 miles north of Blair. He headed south with the South Dakota Police in hot pursuit. When he entered Nebraska, the Nebraska State Patrol took up the pursuit. They never could catch the Firebird. That is one high-powered automobile.

However, as the chase continued down Highway 75, there is a slight curve at the northern edge of the village of Herman that the Firebird failed to negotiate. The car went over a curb, hit a fireplug on the corner and became airborne. The car turned around backward in the air, flew across the street, and landed inside the Sunday school room of the church on that corner. It is fortunate that this did not occur four hours later on this Sunday morning.

When I examined this man in our hospital emergency room, there wasn't a mark on him. He was neurologically intact, except that he was unconscious. His blood alcohol level was near 0.40%—five times today's legal limit of .08%. After about 12 hours of supportive monitoring in our intensive care unit he woke up. He had absolutely no memory of the events of the previous morning. After I informed him of what I knew, he then noticed the police guard standing at the doorway of his hospital room. He then said, "I guess I'm in trouble, aren't I?" Indeed he was.

Over the years I have spent many night-time hours on several occasions struggling with underage teens who had consumed too much alcohol. One such youngster was still a junior high school student. His blood alcohol level was very high. Periodically I had to physically stimulate him to breathe, as the breathing center of his brain was malfunctioning. I was preparing to put him on a ventilator, when things settled down—he survived to see another day.

One soldier at Fort Knox, Kentucky, was not so lucky. I saw him one morning with a blood alcohol level of 0.50%. Sadly, he was dead. He was found in the parking lot of a local bar when the sun came up. One of the first things that I learned in physiology class in medical school was that alcohol kills brain cells. Of course, one may not miss a few million brain cells here, and a few million there, but over the years that adds up. I never have and never will use alcoholic beverages.

THE MAJOR STROKE THAT WAS STOPPED IN ITS TRACKS

AND HOW THE ONGOING AFTERCARE OF THAT EPISODE HELPED PREVENT A FUTURE HEART ATTACK

THE CLOT-BUSTER DRUG, tissue plasminogen activator (tPA), came upon the medical scene in the 1990s. At first tPA was used to dissolve clots in heart vessels, in the lungs and legs. It is interesting to note that the very first use of tPA in Nebraska was right here in Blair.

Dr. Richard Collins, a prominent Omaha cardiologist, attended one of our monthly medical staff meetings, bringing with him some samples of tPA, which had been newly released by the Federal Drug Administration. He had received his first trial samples that very morning, and he wanted to spread the word to as many physicians as possible about this exciting new drug. He had just finished telling us all about tPA when my partner Dr. Grace received a call from our next-door clinic that one of his patients had collapsed in the waiting room. He was rushed across the parking lot on a gurney to our hospital ER with a heart attack in progress. Dr. Collins saw him with Dr. Grace, and they administered that dose of tPA. The patient survived.

The use of tPA in cases of stroke came several years later. For that use the process must be carefully diagnosed and controlled. The first requirement is that it should be started and completed intravenously as soon as possible after the very first onset of stroke symptoms, but no longer than three hours later. The reason for that three-hour window is that brain cells are so fragile that they have little chance of recovery if they are deprived of oxygen any longer than that. The other critical requirement is that, for a stroke, it must be for a clot-induced stroke—not a hemorrhagic stroke. If tPA is given for a stroke caused by a hemorrhaging (bleeding) blood vessel, it will increase the bleeding and may be fatal. Given for a stroke caused by a clot cutting off blood supply, however, tPA may dissolve the clot and be lifesaving. To tell the difference, a special kind of CT scanner is required, a spiral CT scanner. This machine gives the answer almost instantly.

Our medical staff went to our hospital's board of directors and pleaded with them to add this special machine to the radiology department. At first they declined because they said that it was not in our current budget. After we explained to the board that the manufacturer did not charge for the machine outright, but rather charged a fee only for each time that it was used, then the board agreed to acquire one.

The point of this story is that my wife, Carole, was the first one in Blair to receive this new clot buster (tPA) to reverse the symptoms of an impending stroke. Here is her story: One morning in the late 1990s, not long after our new spiral CT scanner had been installed, I got up earlier than normal to get an early start on a busier hospital schedule than usual. As I was heading out the door, my wife and I hugged as usual. As I walked into our hospital ER less than ten minutes later, the ER nurse handed me the telephone and said, "Your wife is on the phone, and I think that you need to talk to her RIGHT NOW!" Carole's speech was slurred, and she was intermittently having trouble moving her right arm and leg, with tingling and numbness in her upper right leg.

Five minutes later I was at her side at home. It only took a few moments for me to decide that I could assist her to my car and have her at our hospital and in the ER long before our local rescue squad could get mobilized. The MD on call for the ER got an IV started while we waited for the results of the spiral CT scan. Within a few minutes we knew that these symptoms were due to a clot in a cerebral blood vessel, and not a bleeding vessel. Immediately the tPA protocol was initiated and completed within the required three-hour window. She was sent directly to Immanuel Hospital in Omaha to see the consulting neurologist. During the thirty-minute ambulance ride, Carole was still having intermittent episodes of right hemiplegia (weakness, tingling and numbness), but reported that these episodes were progressively shorter and less severe. By the time she reached Immanuel Hospital, the episodes had vanished.

A cerebral arteriogram was performed and the neurologist was absolutely amazed that this chain of events, which had threatened to become a full-blown right-sided stroke, resolved with no evidence of residual damage.

As part of her ongoing treatment, Carole was still taking an anticoagulant in 2004 when she had chest pains that resulted in quadruple coronary artery bypass surgery. I believe the fact that she was already taking anticoagulant medicines prior to her heart surgery was a major reason that she had only angina pectoris (chest pain), and not a myocardial infarction (heart attack) before the heart vessel surgery. The events preceding her coronary bypass surgery are detailed elsewhere in this book.

ORANGES AND EGGS: MEMORIES OF DR. RUDOLPH SCHENKEN

DR. SCHENKEN WAS the chair of the Department of Pathology at Nebraska Methodist Hospital in Omaha. He was a prominent physician in our state and nationally. He was well respected and an excellent lecturer. I shall never forget this particular lecture: Dr. Schenken was standing and speaking from behind a long table topped with a lectern. He showed a slide on the screen, in which the surgeon was removing a large tumor. He asked one of my classmates, "How big is that tumor?" My classmate replied, "About the size of an orange." There was a prolonged silence. Then Dr. Schenken turned and retrieved from under the lectern a large grocery sack, which he emptied onto the table. Many oranges of all different sizes rolled onto and off of the table. Amid the laughter, Doctor Schenken said, in a very dominating voice, "Now, doctor, which size orange did you have in mind?" His point, of course, was that we have to learn to be precise.

About three years later during my internship at the Nebraska Methodist Hospital, we interns on the surgical service were gathered at our Saturday morning conference with Dr. Schenken. We presented and discussed the surgical cases in which we were involved during the previous week. I was describing an osteochondroma (a benign cartilaginous tumor) that I had removed from a patient's hand. I mentioned that it was "about the size of a chicken egg." I realized my error before the last word got out of my mouth. I never knew that there were so many different breeds of chickens in this world. I would swear that Dr. Schenken mentioned every single one of them. Again, be precise!

PERCEPTIONS ABOUT THE PRACTICE OF MEDICINE OVER THE SPAN OF MY CAREER

HAS THE NATURE of the practice of medicine really changed over the last 50 years? The short answer is: Yes and No.

YES—the horse and buggy days are gone, thanks to the technology that evolved from the race to the moon and the space age that has evolved since. The nature of the things that doctors are now able to diagnose and do has literally exploded, with all of the digital scans and advances in surgery, medicines and chemotherapies for malignancies that the digital age has made possible.

YES—The depression era is gone (at least for now). The bread and soup kitchen lines have been reduced, but not totally eliminated. Doctor bills are no longer paid with chickens and bushels of sweet corn and fresh tomatoes delivered on their doorsteps by grateful patients. However, in the first two or three decades that I practiced at the Blair Clinic, it was not unusual to have a local farmer or gardener give us a bushel or two of sweet corn or tomatoes at the back door of the clinic with a note to help ourselves.

Now however, the medical professionals are paid by third parties—the government and insurance firms. But in my opinion, each of the third parties pads their own pockets with as much of the money as they can, as the money passes through their hands. Costs have skyrocketed to the point that there seems to be no way that the average Jane or Joe can manage.

YES—The hours that doctors work are vastly different; gone for the most part are the punishing 24/7 workloads. I personally think we owe a debt of gratitude to changes in society. In my lifetime women have taken their place in the medical professions, and both men and women have benefited from changes that have come with that. The responsibilities of the medical profession and parenthood are not really compatible with that 24/7 mindset of old. Family must always take a high priority, and that remains a delicate balance. However, it does take more doctors and/or physicians assistants to do the same amount of work that fewer of us did in the old days. When you add in the additional time demanded of practitioners for computerized record keeping, these two factors contribute to the increase in the total cost of medical care.

YES—we have a more affluent society now than we did over 50 years ago. The odds are that that affluence will not continue forever.

YES—a large number of younger physicians are now employees of a hospital-based system. One of the advantages of such a system is that the doctors no longer have to concern themselves with the day-to-day management details of operating a medical office, such as providing for office space and furnishings, salaries for employees, malpractice insurance, health insurance and retirement benefits, and a long list of items that we at the Blair Clinic had to provide for ourselves. Current Docs and PAs should remember that we old guys did all of that in an era in which the average office call was in the range of five to eight dollars and the total obstetrical fee for the doctor was one hundred twenty-five dollars, including pre and post-natal care as well as the normal delivery itself.

During my first year in Blair, in 1964, the annual bill for my malpractice insurance was in the three- to four-hundred dollar range. Now all the employed doctors have contracts for management of all of those details. I started at the Blair Clinic on the basis of a handshake and three empty rooms—and the opportunity to begin working with a fine, well-respected group of physicians.

YES—The rigidity of computerized medical records systems required for data mining compromises the face-to-face time with the patient. Those factors are forcing many doctors to throw in the towel and retire early.

I recently talked with a new emergency room physician who had previously practiced family medicine much as I have described in this book. He lived in a small town in the middle of Nebraska. The complicated world of computer control which has engulfed medical record keeping caused him to change course to emergency medicine. No wonder that the American Association of Medical Colleges has recently predicted the United States will be short 40,000 to 100,000 physicians by 2030.

NO—The focus on the individual doctor-patient relationship has—and must—continue. From the days of Hippocrates and Jesus over 2500 years ago and counting, that has never changed. Even the interference of government and the corporate administration of medicine must not, and WILL not, change that focus.

All of the above being said, I still feel that the practice of medicine is the best profession in the world. One can do no better than to devote one's life to the healing professions.

FINAL COMMENTS

THESE FINAL COMMENTS are mostly directed to those readers who are in, or entering, the medically-related professions. However, these principles apply equally to everyone. For most of the years during the last decade of my career, I was invited by the family practice department of the University of Nebraska College of Medicine to give the final lecture to their third-year residents. The core message of that lecture was, "Take care of yourselves—you will not do your patients any good if you are dead." I also urged them to be sure that they take regular vacations in order to get away from it all for a few days to prevent burn-out.

Here is a suggestion for the new doctors: when you first start your new practice, find yourself experienced nurses and then do as they advise. That will help the transition to your new world of practicing medicine. I also suggested that everyone in your family, including yourself, should have their own personal physician. However, that does become more of a challenge if you are in a rural area.

Here is another nugget, for doctors of any age. When a patient says to you, as you have your hand on the doorknob as you are leaving the room, "By the way, Doc..." —then stop, turn around and listen. The message very possibly is the reason for their visit in the first place.

This happened to me once many years ago. As I put my hand on the doorknob, the patient asked me if I would look into an ear that had been bothering him. So, I reached for my otoscope that was hanging on the wall behind him. The ear canal contained a large, slightly raised, shiny and very black mole which was obviously a malignant melanoma. Because of its almost inaccessible location, I did not even attempt to biopsy it myself. Instead I immediately sent him to a head and neck surgeon. The next time that I had a chance to see him in my office, over a year or two later, he was sporting a very realistic facial prosthetic device which included almost the entire side of his face, and the lower one half of the ear on that side of his head. To that point the surgery looked like it had controlled his malignancy. I lost contact with him since. I wish I had been able to hear of the long-term result.

Closer to home, at some point as you are hurrying out of the house to get an early start, you will be asked to check one of your family members. It's important to stop and assess the situation - and always be aware of your family's medical history. For instance, my wife Carole's own family experienced significant medical issues resulting in birth defects with cardiac anomalies, and career-ending premature deaths due to cardiovascular disease.

One evening in the winter of 2004, Carole decided to go for a walk. After a half block it started to snow, so she turned and climbed back up the rather steep hill. She sat down in the chair beside me and said, "Coming back up the hill, I had this squeezing pain in the middle of my chest, but it is gone now, and I feel fine." I checked her pulse and listened to her heart and said, "Dr. Collins will be at our hospital at 8 a.m. tomorrow for his routine cardiac clinic. Let's meet him there."

The next morning Dr. Collins put her on the treadmill for a cardiac stress test. After only a minute or two, he said "Stop." I was watching over his shoulder and immediately saw what he meant by that remark. There were marked S-T segment changes in every lead on the EKG. The heart muscles were not getting enough oxygen during exercise due to multiple partially clogged arteries.

He promptly sent Carole directly to Immanuel Hospital in Omaha for "protective custody" for the weekend, and scheduled a cardiac catheterization for Monday morning. On Tuesday morning she underwent a quadruple coronary artery bypass procedure. Fortunately, there was no indication of any cardiac muscle damage. A heart attack had been prevented. She still sees her cardiologist on a regular basis, and is doing well.

One of our sons, when he was in his late 40s, had some chest pains while he was climbing a long and steep stairway. He called his own doctor. He had a single-vessel stent placed shortly thereafter and still goes to the cardiologist for regular checkups. The message with all of this—know your own family history. It is essential that you are aware of what could be in store for you.

Dr. Rudy Sievers was one of the original partners in the Blair Clinic. As a new young doctor I really had no idea what to charge patients for my services. Frequently I went to him to discuss what would be an appropriate charge for the service that I had provided. Then one day Rudy said, "Just take good care of your patients, and the money will take care of itself." That proved to be wonderful advice for that era of the practice of medicine. In today's world, with the prevalent corporate model of practice, that attitude is fighting an uphill battle. I will repeat again—almost all doctors today complain that the growing demand for computer data-mining takes more and more time away from the hands-on, face-to-face care of their patients.

A final thought: recalling the events featured in this book makes me realize even more this truth: It has been an honor and a privilege to have been present at some of the most joyous times, as well as some of the times of deepest sorrow, of so many of my patients, friends and neighbors.

As Hippocrates is quoted: "Where the art of medicine is loved, therein lies the love of humanity."

K. C. Bagby, M.D.

www.ingramcontent.com/pod-product-compliance
Lightning Source LLC
Chambersburg PA
CBHW020927180526
45163CB00007B/2908